SANDEEP PALAKODETI, MD, MPH

THE

I0022870

Ultimate
ASSET

A precision
medicine guide
for more years
at your best

EXTEND YOUR PRIME,
NOT JUST YOUR LIFESPAN

The
Ultimate
Asset

*Extend Your Prime,
Not (Just) Your Lifespan*

Sandeep Palakodeti, MD, MPH

This book is for informational purposes only. It is not intended to serve as a substitute for professional medical advice. The author and publisher specifically disclaim any and all liability arising directly or indirectly from the use of any information contained in this book. A healthcare professional should be consulted regarding your specific medical situation. Any product mentioned in this book does not imply endorsement of that product by the author or publisher.

The conversations in the book are based on the author's recollections, though they are not intended to represent word-for-word transcripts. Rather, the author has retold them in a way that communicates the meaning of what was said. In the author's humble opinion, the essence of the dialogue is accurate in all instances.

Velocity Health
203 East Broadway Street, Unit 498
Granville, Ohio 43023
www.velocityhealthclinic.com

Publisher's Cataloging-In-Publication Data

Names: Palakodeti, Sandeep, author.
Title: The ultimate asset : extend your prime, not (just) your lifespan / Sandeep Palakodeti, MD, MPH.
Description: Granville, Ohio : Velocity Health, [2026] | Includes bibliographical references.
Identifiers: ISBN: 9798993924403 (hardcover) | 9798993924410 (softcover) | 9798993924427 (ebook) | 9798993924434 (audiobook)
Subjects: LCSH: Aging--Prevention. | Middle-aged persons--Health and hygiene. | Longevity. | Vitality. | Rejuvenation.
Classification: LCC: RA776.75 .P35 2026 | DDC: 613.2--dc23

"*The Ultimate Asset* is the book the longevity field has been waiting for—clear, actionable, scientifically grounded, and relentlessly focused on what actually improves human healthspan. Dr. Palakodeti translates cutting-edge precision medicine into a roadmap anyone can follow to reclaim energy, prevent chronic disease, and extend the most productive years of life."

— Robert Lufkin, MD, Physician, Professor, and *New York Times* Bestselling Author of *Lies I Taught in Medical School*

"Health is the one asset, the ultimate asset, that underwrites every ambition and fuels every dream. Dr. Palakodeti's book is that rare blend of rigorous science, relatable practices, and relevant examples to help protect, manage, and grow one's health particularly in the latter half of life. I highly recommend this book to anyone who is looking for a sound strategy in place of guesswork or unproven trends to make the most of a healthy life."

— Neeli Bendapudi, PhD

"In *The Ultimate Asset*, Dr. Sandeep Palakodeti brings exceptionally rare credibility to the conversation on longevity and leadership in medicine. Blending rigorous clinical science, hard-earned executive insight, and deep humanity, he reframes healthspan as both a personal responsibility and a societal imperative. This is not aspirational medicine. It is the kind of prescription we need most and need now. It is a clear, disciplined blueprint for extending your prime and redefining modern healthcare."

— Jon Van Der Veer, DO, Founder and CEO, Hy-Vee Health Exemplar Care

"*The Ultimate Asset* is one of the rare longevity books that gets it right. As a women's health and performance physician, I see too many approaches that either oversimplify aging or turn it into an extreme biohacking project. This book offers something far more useful—a grounded, systems-based framework for extending your prime, not just your lifespan.

What stands out is the shift from 'normal for your age' to what's actually possible with personalized, data-driven medicine, especially for women navigating midlife, hormonal change, leadership, and caregiving all at once. The Core Four (sleep, nutrition, movement, mental resilience) are clinically sound, but the deeper value is the emphasis on agency, function, and purpose.

This isn't about chasing youth. It's about building a body and mind capable of carrying your life forward with strength, clarity, and vitality. For women who want to stay sharp, strong, and fully engaged in the second half of life, this book is both practical and deeply empowering."

— Dr. Brittany Busse, Founder and President, Vitel Health Physician Services Cooperative

To Abby, Devin, and Lily

Contents

Velocity Executive Health Briefings To Preserve Your Prime

4 In-Depth Healthspan-Extension Reports – Yours Free

Compliments of Velocity Health Clinic, get instant access to:

www.velocityhealthclinic.com/book-resources

Preface: 50 Is the New 30

Every story has an origin. This is the origin story.

I wrote this book for several reasons. **One**, because it's the book I wish I had as an early clinician. Back then, I was doing what all well-trained physicians are taught to do—follow the guidelines, trust the system, manage illness. What I didn't yet understand was that there's a world beyond "sickcare," a world where the goal isn't to manage disease but to optimize healthspan. If I had had this framework years ago, I would have started much sooner in helping people live better, longer—rather than waiting until symptoms appeared to intervene. I would have recognized that longevity isn't luck. It's literacy. It's learning how to read your own biology, and then writing a better story with it.

Two, every doctor needs a book. What we know best serves the world when it's written down, packaged professionally, and distributed to the masses—not just to our peers within the industry. Medical knowledge locked inside clinics and conferences doesn't transform lives. But a message in print can travel farther, reach wider, and plant the seed of possibility in someone who's ready for change.

And **three**, I wrote this book to offer a path for those aspiring to lengthen their healthspan to make their dreams come true—to live better, longer, as if they were younger—and to make that so. We have the tools, the tests, and the understanding to do this now. The science exists. The question is: *Will we use it?*

Once I decided to write the book, the obvious next question was what to call it. I settled on *The Ultimate Asset* because that's what your healthspan truly is—something to be protected, preserved, and progressed into the future. It's not the luck of genetics. It can be intentional. It can be designed. It can be extended. Your prime can last as long as you need it to. Decline is optional. That's more than some slogan . . . it's a physiological reality waiting to be claimed by anyone who's ready to understand their body differently.

When I founded my concierge healthspan optimization clinic, Velocity Health, this message resonated most with executives and with men. So the previous title was *The Executive Edge*. It fit the spirit of the early days of the company and our innovative clientele—high-performing founders, CEOs, and professionals looking for that extra 5 percent of clarity, energy, and longevity that separates thriving from surviving. To my surprise and delight, it turns out that the message of optimizing one's healthspan resonated particularly strongly with women. In fact, 60 percent of Velocity Health patients are now women and hail from many different professional backgrounds. That single statistic changed how I thought about the message entirely. It revealed that the desire to optimize, to take control, to stay vibrant and capable, is universal. It's not a "biohacker" trend, or a male trend, or an executive trend . . . it's a human one. *The Executive Edge* also left out non-executives and non-founders, the people who carry families, run communities, and influence the health decisions that shape generations.

At the same time, the broader trend toward concierge and precision healthcare was taking shape. The movement was led by upper-middle-class Gen X types—those in their forties and fifties who grew up trusting doctors but now demand more from the system. They are proactive, not reactive. They want comprehensive testing, early diagnostics, and personalized care plans. And they are finding, more and more, that the traditional healthcare system is unprepared for such patients. The system was built for disease management, not for health creation.

For a while, the new working title *50 Is the New 30* captured that energy. It said what people were beginning to believe, which is that midlife no longer has to mean decline, that the vitality of youth can be recaptured—and sustained—for decades. And while it was catchy, it didn't quite fit the full value of what we do at Velocity Health. Feeling younger matters, yes, but more specifically, we're here to help protect, preserve, and prosper what matters most—healthspan.

That's how *The Ultimate Asset* became the final title. It captures everything—the science, the philosophy, and the mission. It's about age reversal and individual optimization and empowerment. It speaks to both genders, all professions, every person who's ready to take ownership of their biology and future. It helps that *The Ultimate Asset* is also the name of the official Velocity Health podcast. That's where my team and I sit down with world-class physicians, health coaches, and high-performing executives (naturally) to cover in longform, deep conversation what it really takes to feel, look, and perform at your best. On the show, we cover it all. And that is what I do in this book. If you'd like that expanded content, check out *The Ultimate Asset* podcast wherever you download or stream your favorite shows.

This book captures succinctly the takeaways of the podcast. And I further distill everything gleaned from those conversations, from Velocity Health, and from the lives already transformed when people finally realize that their healthspan—their vitality, capability, and freedom—isn't fixed . . . it's changeable. Age is a number, but it's not the only number. I'll show you what those numbers are in this book—and how to improve, monitor, and otherwise optimize them.

This is the book that will teach you how to invest in your health so you can keep it for decades to come. In the chapters that follow, I will introduce a disciplined, data-informed, human-centered approach to healthspan that is the antidote to both burnout and biohacking—and is what is needed for society to regain proper function and control. I will ask more of you than the short attention span of a quick fix. But I will give you far more in return, including a way to live in your body with agency instead of anxiety, with clarity instead of confusion, and with a sense that your best years are not a memory but a project under construction. You will encounter not only concepts and frameworks but also real people—Velocity Health patients—whose lives changed when they stopped accepting decline as inevitable. You will encounter these personal stories as case studies that show how we pulled individuals like you out of decline and helped them reclaim strength, presence, and clarity. You will meet executives, parents, caregivers, and midlife strivers who were told they were just getting older—but then discovered what becomes possible when you refuse to accept that as a final verdict. My hope is that as you walk with them through their turning points, through the frightening test results, the sleepless nights, and the small daily decisions that began to compound in their favor, you will start to recognize pieces of your own story. I hope you will feel a quiet but unmistakable conviction that if they can do it, then you can as well. That belief is the promise of *The Ultimate Asset*, and that belief is where our work together begins.

To whet your learning appetite, here are **thirty specific things** this book will teach you:

- **Why this might be your last real window to rescue your healthspan—and how to know if you're already wasting it.**

- How "fine" became the most dangerous four-letter word in modern medicine—and what it's really hiding in your labs.

- **The single conversation with yourself every fiftysomething must have before they ask for more time.**

- How five brutally honest questions can expose the real mission for your second half of life.

- **The surprising reason your grandkids are the most powerful longevity drug there is.**

- Why traditional sickcare keeps telling you, "You're normal for your age"—and how to turn that sentence into a warning siren.

- **The real reason you're exhausted at 3:00 p.m.—and why your midlife comeback starts with sleep, not supplements.**

- How to conduct your own "Sleep Symphony" so hormones, brain, and metabolism finally play the same song.

- **The hidden ways light, temperature, and technology are wrecking your nights—and the simple rituals that flip them in your favor.**

- What one exhausted caregiver taught us about the cruel lie of "just go to bed earlier"—and how she actually got her life back.

- **Why most people's nutrition is *not* a problem because they're undisciplined (it's an issue because no one ever showed them a system like the Velocity Nutrition Strategy).**

- The one primary objective you must choose for your food (and why trying to chase three goals at once keeps you stuck).

- **How a DEXA scan, CGM, and a few smart constraints turned two very different people into nutrition success stories.**

- The restaurant "script set" that lets you eat out, enjoy yourself, and still walk away with your healthspan intact.

- **Why your supplement drawer looks impressive but your results don't—and how midlife-specific guidance finally changes that.**

- The three pillars of fitness that matter far more than the number on your scale after 50.

- **How to pick the right workout protocol—fat loss, metabolic rehab, body recomposition, cognitive energy, gut repair, or cardiac health—so your training actually matches your life.**

- The base weekly structure that lets real people with jobs, kids, and travel still train like they care about the next 30 years.

- **The overlays no one talks about: how medical constraints, hormones, and messy logistics quietly sabotage your workouts—and how to plan around all three.**

- Why some seasons of life feel like they're trying to break you—and how to tell whether you need a new routine or a new system.

- **The three-layer "mental health stack" that turns baseline screening, resilience practices, and social health into a real defense against burnout.**

- How using your mind on purpose—learning, engaging, stretching—may be the cheapest cognitive longevity tool on the planet.

- **The gratitude habit that multiplies the impact of everything else you're doing for your brain and mood.**

- Why an ordinary annual check-up is nowhere near enough—and how an executive-level advanced diagnostic can rewrite your future.

- **The imaging and cardio-fitness tests (like CAC, CCTA, and VO₂ max) that quietly reveal whether you're aging faster than your birth certificate says.**

- The genomic, epigenetic, and bloodwork "deep dive" that turns vague risk into a precise, personalized health plan.

- **The advanced therapeutics decision framework that keeps you from wasting money on trendy interventions that don't move your markers.**

- The naked-honest truth about peptides, rapamycin, PRP, and HBOT—and when they finally make sense after foundations are in place.

- **How concierge support, quarterly reassessment, and a redesigned healthcare system can transform your healthspan into your ultimate asset.**

If even just **three** of these insights in this book—just 10 percent—stick with you, **those alone will change everything**.

That's how transformation works. It starts with a single insight that refuses to leave you alone. It grows quietly until one day you look in the mirror and realize you don't just feel better . . . you **are** better.

So let's begin there. What comes now is what I call the Last Window, that final season of life in which lasting change is still possible. Rescue and improve your healthspan now, in this midlife season, or your prime truly is over. But do it right, and your best days won't be behind you. They'll still be ahead . . . waiting to be lived.

Introduction: The Last Window

One in five patients discharged from the number-one hospital in the world comes back within thirty days due to complications. I know because I chaired that very hospital's readmission committee. But it wasn't just us; a 20 percent readmission rate was historically standard across US healthcare.[1] I remember thinking, *We're the best hospital in the world and we can't fix this? That's insane.*

That moment came after decades of personal and professional experiences that shaped how I now see health, medicine, and human wellness—and why I came to believe the entire system needs a complete reset.

Within my family, there was a cruel irony.

As a youngster, I wasn't thinking about healthcare policy or systemic reform. I lifted weights, played recreational hockey and pickup football with my friends, swam every summer, hiked most weekends, and generally loved the outdoors. I was more active than athletic, if that makes sense. I was just trying to stay fit, have fun, and really . . . make the best of what I'd later realize was an unhelpful health substrate. My family's South Asian genetics were stacked against us; metabolic syndrome ran rampant. Back in our ancestral home, our diet and health culture are suboptimal, so staying in shape felt like an uphill climb both ways, so to speak. For years, I couldn't figure out why. When my parents resettled in a quaint suburban town in Ohio, USA, they adopted many aspects of Midwest American culture: food choices, daily activities, and lifestyle priorities. My father was a physician; my brother became a physician as well. We had all the knowledge and resources in the world to be our absolute healthiest. But that didn't mean we could stop our grandparents from dying in their sixties from heart attacks. As for my dad, he has had multiple heart attacks himself. I remember rushing to the hospital . . . keeping vigil by his bedside . . . wondering if one day it would be my turn to lay in a bed just like that, surrounded by family . . . feeling this way. This terrible, horrible, powerless way.

There's more. Type-2 diabetes also runs in the family (both of my parents). And my brother developed diabetes briefly but was able to reverse it. I knew my genetics were not doing my health any favors, and I was doing everything I could to stay active in school up through premed—but every man in my family would suffer the same fate if not for immense intervention.

The realization didn't hit me until I finished my residency, when I reached my absolute unhealthiest, a far cry from my prior life, when I was much more active. The irony of being a newly minted physician was that I had, at the same time, let myself slide into the most unhealthy period of my life. I weighed 250 pounds, was pre-diabetic, had lost my hair, fell under circadian distress, ate poorly, stayed stressed, and couldn't sleep.

My brother and I were born in the United Kingdom after my parents moved there from India, but then our family moved to Ohio. Growing up, I remember (as much as I can) how my parents had to decide which parts of our previous South Asian culture to keep and which aspects to assimilate into American culture. For example, do you go out for pizza and burgers with friends, or keep eating traditional foods? The South Asian diet is very high in carbs and starch, low in protein, and high on the glycemic index—a recipe for insulin resistance. There's not much emphasis on physical activity or exercise in India; instead, there's more focus on education and book smarts. Health wasn't a cultural priority; your health was something that "just happened" while you lived your life. Some got lucky, others not so much.

Now, when I compare the high-carb, low-fat, low-protein Indian diet to the Standard American Diet (also known as "SAD"), both are terrible in different ways. At least in my upbringing, my mom cooked fresh food every day. We grew a lot of our own vegetables, went to the farmer's market, and ate real, whole foods. But the meals were still heavy on carbs and starch, with little protein. Even when you compare something like a curry with brown rice and chickpeas as the protein source—maybe with some tofu added—it's still relatively low in protein. The sauce might be a fresh, minimally processed blend of spices and greens. It's healthy in the sense that it's fresh and whole, but protein is low. Compare that to a hamburger—especially fast food—which is ultra-processed, made with bleached, enriched white flour, but still contains about four times more protein. For my parents, the novelty of Pizza Hut, Burger King, and other fast food chains were all a part of assimilating.

At school, I never felt self-conscious about lunch. My parents packed lunches that fit in from time to time—a PB&J sandwich, potato chips—or let us get the pizza and burgers most public schools feed students. At home, my mom made fresh, home-cooked meals. The difference was stark: fresh, whole foods at home that were still low in protein, contrasted with the processed, high-protein American foods outside. I was constantly navigating between the two, always seeking better options but bumping up against the Standard American Diet.

Into adolescence, I continued to stay recreationally active. I also picked up tennis and played rugby. Also, I played golf. Rugby wasn't offered at Beavercreek High School, so I sought it out separately, playing with the Wright State University club team while I was still in high school, then continuing into college. I attended the University of Dayton for undergraduate, then back to Wright State for a master's in public health and medical school.

Coming out of college, I was at a healthy weight, felt great, and felt at a peak in my early twenties, the physical prime of life. Medical school has a way of slowly wearing you down, but I could still maintain my health as a student because I had some flexibility. Residency, though, is what breaks you. Your schedule is not your own. You're told to be somewhere for twelve straight hours, with little control over your time. You prepare for those shifts, decompress from them, and then do it all over again. You pull nonstop thirty-six-hour shifts without realizing how much broken sleep damages your health. Ironically, I violated nearly every principle I now teach—sleep, nutrition, stress management, for example—while training to prevent the very conditions that lifestyle creates. Residency completely wrecks your biology, and it stacks up year after year. So do the extra pounds.

Even so, I completed a fellowship at Harvard Medical School and was on staff at Mayo. I maintained a strong belief that I should do something bigger than myself. Growing up, I'd always felt there are a few areas where most people can make the greatest impact in the short time we have, those being education, intelligence, and health. Health was for me. But not just the industry as it was but as it could be. Since college, I've believed that we are about to enter a health-tech age where we have no idea what the end of life will look like for many of us. Twenty or thirty years from now, I truly think people will be living to 120 or 130 years of age. That will change everything, from relationships to careers to entitlements to, yes, healthcare. Staying at the forefront of the future, exploring it intellectually, was a path I found through science in high school—biology, specifically. I wanted to understand the limits of the human body and mind and where they might go in decades and centuries to come. Healing people, helping people, and connecting with them one-on-one through that lens is something I still love every day. My motivation then and now is to create a system that allows as many people as possible to thrive well into the future and see whatever the next phase of humanity will be. That's why that opening moment at the hospital hit me so hard. Even at the pinnacle of my profession, I could see the cracks in the foundation.

Ivy League-trained, board-certified, and fast-tracked to the top of corporate medicine, I had checked every box of what my profession calls "success." I worked at a leading hospital. I helped build value-based care models across the country. I became an executive at one of the largest health insurers in America. From the outside, it looked like I was shaping the future of medicine.

But on the inside, my stomach churned. Our healthcare system is *not* designed to keep people well. It's structured to keep money flowing. You see, hospitals profit from readmissions, insurers profit from premiums and denials, pharmaceutical companies profit from lifelong customers, and even policymakers profit from keeping the game going. Everyone has their hand in the till, and the cash-grab lives off human sickness.

I cannot, however, blame any one individual or even group. I did my best, as the overwhelming majority of healthcare professionals, specialists, support staff, and administrators do. Yet no amount of goodwill can overcome bad design. The incentives are so deeply misaligned that the system actively promotes illness *despite* the good hearts of those involved. Doctors are chained to RVUs, billing codes, and throughput quotas. Patients are reduced to "covered lives" on a spreadsheet. Executives celebrate "cost savings" while quality metrics stagnate or decline. And through it all, families like mine—genetically vulnerable, culturally at risk, doing our best to be healthy—are crushed in the gears of a machine that prioritizes profit over prosperity.

I can't fix a system like that from within. In Ohio growing up, I often heard the expression, "If it ain't broke, don't fix it." The unspoken corollary to that might be something like, "If it's definitely broke, don't fix it; start over."

That's the conclusion my healthcare journey brought me to. The system wasn't simply broken and in need of patches, repairs, and greasing; it was *made* this way. Incremental reform was never going to work. We need factory recall. Metaphorically speaking, that's what I did—I smashed the reset button.

I pivoted to value-based care, then to building new care models nationwide. But eventually I realized something: Incremental reform doesn't work. We need a whole new system. That's why I would go on to found **Velocity Health** (www.velocityhealthclinic. com). I believe in a renewed vision for medicine, one that is rooted in empathy, fueled by scientific rigor, and committed to unleashing the fullest expression of who you as an individual are. Velocity provides an "escape velocity" from the status quo, from a potentially disappointing lifespan and even shorter healthspan, and into a life of vitality and vigor.

Velocity Health blows up the current "sickcare" paradigm of healthcare and starts fresh. Consider this question: If you were to create a clinical model we would want for ourselves and our families, what would that look like? Certainly it would be personalized, proactive, and with interdisciplinary care that wraps around you, the patient. The new model would help prevent chronic disease from starting, would promote wellness, and find disease early enough to stamp it out before it became a problem. It would operate outside of the traditional health insurance system, which has handcuffed physicians into practicing a certain way, following guidelines and regulations that often go against their professional expertise and what's right for patients. The new system would encourage patients to protect themselves with catastrophic insurance and indemnity insurance for unforeseen events. But ultimately, the focus would be on keeping people as healthy as possible in this new paradigm.

The difference between the new model at Velocity Health and the traditional one starts with what the average patient experiences today. In the US, the average primary care visit is seven minutes long. Physicians interrupt their patients within thirty seconds of them speaking. Most patients see their doctor between zero and four times a year—most often zero or one—so there's no real relationship, no true trust. Meanwhile, physicians themselves may have informal networks, colleagues they can text to ask, "I know the guideline says this, but what do you actually think?" The keyword is *may*; this varies provider to provider. Yours may—or may not.

Deeply personalized care isn't available to most people because the system is designed around "relative value units" (RVUs), which tie physicians' pay to the number of billable services they perform. To keep up, doctors are forced to churn through as many RVUs as possible just to pay off med school debt and maintain their high-status, high-budget lifestyle out in their community. Patients feel that rush and that transactional energy, and so do the doctors. Everyone feels like a widget in a machine. They are.

Velocity is the opposite of all of it. We spend time with our patients. We don't manage thousands of names on a panel; we have a couple hundred. We know their names, their spouses' names, their kids' names, their dogs' names, what they do for a living, their culture, what kind of food they enjoy, and what kind they don't. Many of these stories we have memorized because we consider these people our extended family. We often meet in person. We share a history.

This is what I love about medicine the Velocity way; we pair a deep understanding of a person's life and our knowledge of human nature with the complexity of educated decision-making. Even in an age of artificial intelligence (AI), where technology may get diagnosis and treatment suggestions exactly right, there will always be multiple options for every medical finding. Choosing the right one depends on truly knowing the patient's context.

We've had some powerful results at Velocity Health along these lines. In one case, we found thyroid cancer in a thirty-five-year-old because we ran the extra testing protocols that Velocity uses, testing that wouldn't happen in a traditional primary care office. In another, we identified leukemia in a man in his thirties not because of exotic testing but because we had the time to notice and question a persistent abnormality on his lab results— low platelets for five years. His previous doctor had dismissed it. We asked the right questions, investigated further, and caught it at stage one.

While it's unfortunate for anyone to face those

diagnoses, the happy ending is that we caught them early enough to change the trajectory of their lives. That's why Velocity exists—to mitigate risk upstream, find problems early, address even minute concerns, and keep our people living better, longer. We go deep into the data and follow where it leads.

Which brings us to this book, *The Ultimate Asset.* As the title indicates, this is written for a specific population, one which we tend to see at Velocity Health more commonly than any other. I want to reach more midlife professionals than we can handle as one-on-one clients at Velocity. The late forties through early sixties, this decade-and-a-half set of years, is the last window for change most people have. Especially for men and women in positions of leadership—in business, in government, in the community, even in your own personal life—the window doesn't slide down. The higher the life stress, the faster it gets slammed shut.

Regardless of your background, the fact of midlife remains: That health-change window is closing fast. For too many—like my grandparents—it slammed shut and never reopened. Miss your moment, and you'll miss the active, fulfilling future you could have had.

CHAPTER 1
Concierge Precision Medicine

What is a good day? For most people, it's a day with energy, vitality, joy, meaning, satisfaction. It's professional success and personal fulfillment. There's running the show and also kicking back. A job well done but also leisure time in solitude and peace, or perhaps quality moments with those you love. You look pretty good, feel great, and, without question, are physically capable of doing what you want.

By the time you're in your fifties, you have 500 such good days left, if that—good being, *I feel good today. Just . . . really good.* You know how it feels to feel good. No complaints. Just good. Very good.

But by age sixty, the number is down to the double digits for most people. After that, for ten, fifteen, sometimes twenty years, there are no good days anymore. That's when you fill your day with adult daycare-like activities to busy yourself so you don't feel as if you're waiting to die. All the while, assisted living, nursing care, or in-home help spend down your savings until you reach poverty and government assistance kicks in for the rest of your natural life. Nothing is left for your kids or grandkids.

This is the default for **most people**. Now, not everyone is resigned to suffer such a fate. In fact, you might have already corrected me in your head by calling to mind such-and-such actress, celebrity athlete, or other entertainer who's living large and looking their best well into the golden years. Such influencers perpetually display their energy and tout their remarkable midlife beauty. What's their secret? How are the rich and famous living their best life while so many others are left counting the years till the end? Is it more than plastic surgery and hormone replacement therapy? What's the secret?

Allow me to expose it, all of it. Three words describe what high-performers know and do that normal people don't: **concierge precision medicine**. It goes like this:

- *concierge* = personalized, high-touch service

- *precision* = no guesswork, no generic "average patient" approach, just your unique data

- *medicine* = the practice of restoring and sustaining health

Notice how this differs from one-size-fits-all medicine, where there is one right thing to eat, one right way to exercise, one right way to manage any symptoms and prevent or reverse a given chronic disease. Scientific studies are valuable, but at the end of the day, **n=1**. Each person's health is its own experiment, and no single intervention affects everyone the same way. What works wonders for one person may fall flat for another. That's why you—yes, you, specifically—need a systematic approach tailored to your own unique biology. Something that reveals what actually works for you, not some generic average patient that doesn't exist.

Consider the rich and famous from earlier. We celebrate these as the healthiest among us, of course. Why are they so? Concierge precision medicine. How they do anything is how they do everything. Private chef, personal trainer, concierge precision healthcare. It just makes sense. They live long and live well because of concierge precision medicine. Because they understand something very important.

Nothing works for everyone. But some things work for some people. I wrote this book to help you discover your "something" so you can reclaim your vitality and unlock the capacity to live long and live well for many more years than you otherwise might have.

What if you could live, and lead, as if you were thirty again—but this time with the wisdom, leverage, and authority of your fifties and sixties?

That is the question I have set out to answer; the major part of the solution is what I call the **Core Four framework**. These are sleep, nutrition, movement, and mental resilience. Aging is guaranteed; aging out of your active lifestyle is optional. Together with the Core Four, I'm going to show you how to integrate cutting-edge diagnostics and recovery protocols that rebuild the function of your youth from the cellular level up. Consider this book your precise, physician-guided strategy for becoming sharper, stronger, and more influential over the next two to three decades. Consider the following Velocity Health patients whose stories may resemble yours.

In this book, we'll walk you through the Core Four. Along the way, you won't need gimmicks or longevity fads. What you need is a clear framework, ruthless self-awareness, and a systems-level protocol that aligns your physiology with your ambitions. That's exactly what this book gives you: the playbook, and the tools to implement it with precision.

The Proof Is in the Proof

The following stories are all based on real Velocity Health Clinic patients; names and other identifying details have changed to protect anonymity. That said, these are the sorts of transformative stories you can expect to model your own after. Because when you do what works better, as these individuals have done, you get better results. That's what we want for you.

So, let's what Velocity Health may be able to do for you via the counsel you'll be receiving from this very book. Starting with . . .

A 52-year-old CFO named **James** came to us burned out, with labs in the "normal" range and no clinical diagnosis. Within three months, we identified silent insulin resistance, sleep apnea, low muscle mass, and early coronary calcification. Today, James is lifting again, sleeping through the night, and has even told us he feels like he's "back in his thirties." This system works because it's built for precision and not platitudes

on getting old, missing out, and losing yourself.
Brian, a 49-year-old CEO from Oregon, was a high-powered executive who suddenly felt twice his age. Long work hours and constant stress had led him to gain weight, sleep poorly, and lose the energetic edge he once had. Traditional doctors brushed off his complaints because his basic check-up numbers were "fine," leaving him frustrated that he felt rundown despite doing "everything right" on paper. At Velocity Health, we took an all-encompassing approach, spending several hours listening to his history and ordering comprehensive labs and screenings that went far beyond the standard. Those tests uncovered the real issues: early insulin resistance, a borderline thyroid imbalance, mild sleep apnea, and cortisol levels that were sky-high from chronic stress—problems his seven-minute annual physical had never caught. With this data, we built a personalized plan: optimizing his nutrition by cutting late-night carb snacking at business dinners and adding more protein, instituting a strict sleep routine to address apnea, and teaching him stress-management strategies like mindfulness breaks during the workday and evening walks to decompress. Over the next year, the transformation was dramatic. The weight came off, his labs normalized—fasting insulin dropped—and his energy returned. He began lifting again, sleeping through the night, and says he feels healthier at 49 than he did at 39. "Dr. Deep did more for my health in one year than all my other doctors combined," he said.

Sarah, 45, a tech CEO and mom, exemplifies the squeezed middle-aged professional balancing a demanding job and a family. By the time she found Velocity Health, she had been feeling chronically off—low energy, trouble concentrating, and mood swings—even though she exercised and tried to eat healthy. She confided, "I just didn't feel my normal self," but every time she got a workup her doctors told her, "This is just part of getting older," and sent her on her way. In our extended consultation she admitted she was struggling to sleep through the night and felt drained in the afternoons. We ordered a comprehensive hormone panel and micronutrient testing alongside full bloodwork, and sure enough, her results explained her puzzling symptoms: early perimenopause with shifting estrogen and progesterone levels causing fatigue and brain fog, a subclinical thyroid slowdown that sapped her energy and mood, and low ferritin, signaling borderline iron deficiency. With these insights, we built Sarah a personalized plan, optimizing her diet for iron and protein, adding gentle thyroid and hormone support, creating a strict wind-down routine to improve her sleep, and coaching her on stress management, ultimately suggesting she delegate more at work and practice morning meditation. Within a few months, she no longer crashed in the afternoons; her energy was steady all day. Sarah's story proves that "normal" labs don't always mean healthy. By digging deeper into her biology, we helped her feel ten years younger, reclaim her stride as both an executive and a mom, and maintain the balance she thought was gone.

Linda, 54, a business owner, had spent decades building her company, but by her mid-50s she feared she was losing her edge. Brain fog, belly weight, and erratic sleep left her exhausted, while menopause symptoms—hot flashes and mood swings—disrupted her days. Her gynecologist offered standard hormone replacement, but Linda wanted a more nuanced approach. At Velocity Health, we confirmed she was indeed in menopause with estrogen and progesterone levels near zero. We also uncovered compounding issues: early osteopenia and elevated cortisol from nonstop stress. We optimized her hormones with carefully monitored bioidentical therapy, adjusted her diet to include more protein and calcium for muscle and bone health, introduced resistance training to rebuild strength, and taught stress-lowering strategies like short yoga routines and scheduled evening downtime. Within six months, Linda's sharpness returned, her metabolism picked up, and she slimmed down—proving midlife weight gain wasn't irreversible. Her sleep deepened, her mood stabilized, and even her bone density began to improve on follow-up scans.

Robert, 59, a financial executive, had always prided himself on being in control, but his father's fatal heart attack at 60 haunted him as he approached that same age. Though he felt fine, his doctor's "okay for now" reassurance wasn't enough, so Robert came to Velocity for a preventive deep dive. Our advanced cardiovascular risk assessment included LDL particle analysis, Lipoprotein(a), and a Coronary Artery Calcium scan followed by CCTA. The results were sobering: His CAC score was elevated for his age and unstable soft plaque was present, despite decent cholesterol numbers.

His Lp(a) was high, explaining his hidden risk. We built a comprehensive prevention plan—heart-healthy nutrition rich in vegetables, fiber, and lean protein; a tailored fitness program with guided cardio intervals; and a high-potency, multi-drug therapy plus omega-3s to stabilize plaque. One year later, his repeat scan showed no progression of disease, his blood pressure and weight were down, and he had lost fifteen pounds. Most importantly, Robert no longer lives under the shadow of his father's fate. Prevention works when you act before the crisis.

Samantha, 50, a wellness blogger, had tried every health trend—intermittent fasting, keto, gut cleanses—and her readers loved following along, but she secretly felt no better. Despite constant hacks, she still had mid-afternoon crashes, and her metabolic markers were trending worse. Frustrated, she joined Velocity Health for expert guidance. We quickly saw the problem: She was overconsuming information. Comprehensive labs, a DEXA scan, and a continuous glucose monitor (CGM) study revealed the truth. Her "healthy" morning smoothie spiked her blood sugar, her cortisol curve was abnormal from poor sleep, and her DEXA showed hidden visceral fat despite her slim frame. We built a Precision Nutrition Plan—protein-rich breakfasts, more fiber, steady sleep times—and taught her stress-calming practices. The results freed her. She had steady energy all day, improved insulin sensitivity, visceral fat trimmed away, and a cortisol rhythm back on track. For the first time, Samantha found joy in simplicity. Her blog shifted too—she began sharing the power of doing what actually works, not chasing the latest fad.

David, 45, an engineer and DIY biohacker, prided himself on self-experiments, from off-label peptides to online testosterone boosters. But he began experiencing unpredictable swings in mood and energy that no spreadsheet could explain. At Velocity, we discovered why: his liver enzymes were elevated from questionable supplements, his "testosterone booster" had suppressed his natural hormone levels, and his heavy-metal screen showed mildly elevated lead. We hit reset: stopping risky compounds, prescribing safe bioidentical hormone therapy under monitoring, and guiding him through a detox protocol. We fine-tuned his supplement stack, focusing only on evidence-backed nutrients. Within weeks, David's mood stabilized and crashes disappeared; within three months, labs confirmed restored balance. Still a biohacker at heart, David now pairs his love of data with medical oversight—finally confident that his experiments are safe and effective.

Nina, 55, a retired executive, wasn't sick—she wanted to future-proof her health. Having watched her mother suffer from dementia, she wanted to avoid that fate. At Velocity, we ran genomic testing and cognitive assessments. Results showed she carried one copy of APOE4, raising her Alzheimer's risk, and her homocysteine was mildly elevated, likely from suboptimal B vitamins. We built a precision brain health plan: a Mediterranean-style diet rich in greens, nuts, and omega-3s; targeted B-vitamin. supplementation; gentle intermittent fasting; and brain-stimulating activities like dance classes, puzzles, and social engagement. Nina embraced it. Her homocysteine dropped to optimal, her energy sharpened, and she even took up learning a new language. Rather than fearing her genes, she's tackling them head-on with a "personal user's manual" for her future.

Oliver, 62, an "extreme" biohacker, was known for trying every new life-extension trick—metformin for longevity, NMN for NAD+ boost, stem-cell infusions, and so on. But he felt winded when on stairs and noticed his grip strength fading. At Velocity, we ran advanced blood tests, VO_2 max, and strength assessments. The results were clear: despite his high-tech hacks, his aerobic capacity was below average, he had lost leg muscle, and his IGF-1 was low, likely from heavy metformin use. We shifted his focus back to fundamentals: pausing unnecessary drugs, building aerobic base with Zone 2 cardio, and adding resistance training. We guided his supplements and introduced supervised NAD+ therapy. Within a year, Oliver's VO_2 max rose 20 percent, his strength returned, and his everyday fitness improved dramatically. He still enjoys cutting-edge science, but now with a foundation that makes it work.

Karen, 45, a working mom of three, had always put her family first and herself last. Exhausted, forgetful, and 20 pounds heavier, she chalked it up to age until Velocity uncovered the truth: hypothyroidism from Hashimoto's, plus vitamin D and iron deficiencies. We started thyroid hormone support, corrected her nutrients, and gave her simple, family-friendly meal strategies and short at-home workouts. Within months, her energy rebounded, her weight began to drop, and even her kids joined in her new yoga routine. Karen's fog lifted, her mood brightened, and she finally realized that caring for herself wasn't selfish—it made her a better mom and role model.

Daniel, 40, a new dad, came in carrying 30 pounds of "sympathy weight" and a pre-diabetes warning from his clinic visit. Busy with career and family, he admitted he had no idea how to start. Our tests confirmed insulin resistance, but also that it was reversible. We built a practical plan: meal-prepped bowls instead of takeout, a CGM to show him real-time blood sugar spikes, and 20-minute home workouts plus family walks. Six months later, Daniel had lost 25 pounds, reversed his pre-diabetes, and regained stamina to play with his toddler and support his wife with a newborn. He said it felt like hitting a reset button—and this time, it's a lifestyle he can sustain.

Laura, 50, a caregiver and mom, had spent years looking after her teens and her aging father, but by the time she reached Velocity she was running on fumes. Severe insomnia left her unrested, her joints ached, and she worried she was slowing down. Tests showed flipped cortisol rhythms, early osteoarthritis, and muscle loss. We focused first on restoring sleep—a dark, cool bedroom, no electronics before bed, magnesium supplementation, journaling, and breathing exercises. For her joints, we paired her with a coach who gave her short daily strength and stretching sessions, and adjusted her diet to be anti-inflammatory with more omega-3s and fewer processed snacks. After weeks of small improvements, Laura hit a milestone—seven hours of total sleep with two of those being deep sleep, her first real nightly rest in years. With energy returning, she built consistency in exercise and nutrition, and her joint pain eased. Three months later, she joined a yoga class, finding joy for herself again. Laura learned that self-care was not selfish but essential, and her renewed calm energy made her more present for her family.

Steven, 55, a devoted father, ignored his health until a colleague's sudden heart attack jolted him awake. With teenagers at home and a family history of heart disease—his father died at 58—Steven came to Velocity anxious but determined. Tests revealed elevated blood pressure, a high Coronary Calcium score, and an unfavorable LDL particle count. We built a prevention strategy: cutting fast food and sodium, adding antioxidant-rich foods, launching a cardio and strength program, and optimizing ApoB with a medication strategy given his risk. Over the next year, Steven lost 20 pounds, normalized his blood pressure, and stabilized his plaque buildup. Now he plays basketball with his son without gasping for breath and feels relief knowing he's broken the cycle that nearly cost him his life.

Michelle, 38, a busy mom and entrepreneur, seemed to have it all together but secretly battled anxiety, mood swings, racing thoughts at night, headaches, and digestive flare-ups. Her labs revealed high cortisol, low B12 and magnesium, and gut dysbiosis. We rebuilt her foundations: replenishing nutrients, correcting gut balance, adding probiotics and fiber, and implementing simple mindfulness practices, including a 10-minute meditation and strict "no emails after 8 p.m." rule.

Exercise was reframed as a mood tool—daily walks and a weekly boxing class. Within weeks, Michelle felt calmer, headaches eased, digestion normalized, and her creativity sparked new ideas for her business. Most importantly, she laughed and played more with her children. Michelle discovered that resilience in mind and body go hand-in-hand, and when both are supported, every part of life benefits.

Eric, 45, a competitive athlete, thought he was invincible. But Velocity's deep dive revealed otherwise: mild arterial plaque, elevated LDL particles, high inflammation markers, and lower-than-ideal testosterone after years of intense training. We tweaked his nutrition to add omega-3s and antioxidants, improved his cardio programming with more Zone 2 work, and adjusted his training schedule for recovery. We also addressed hormone support naturally with sleep and targeted supplements. Months later, Eric noticed faster recovery, better race results, and normalized labs. Even elite performers can have hidden risks, but catching them early meant Eric could continue excelling, not just on the outside but on the inside too.

Sonia, 37, a marathon runner, thought her fatigue was from training until our screenings uncovered a small thyroid tumor. Bloodwork flagged subtle changes, and ultrasound confirmed early thyroid cancer. We connected her with specialists who removed the nodule quickly, essentially curing the cancer at stage 1. After surgery, we carefully balanced her thyroid hormone replacement and guided her recovery with nutrition and mental health support. Within months, Sonia was back to running—

and faster than before—grateful that proactive testing caught a silent danger early. She now tells friends that being proactive about health is as important as training plans, proof that early detection saves lives.

Mark, 50, a former college football player, was still active but carried old injuries, extra weight, and daily aches. His scans showed knee arthritis, shoulder inflammation, low muscle mass, and visceral fat driving inflammation. Instead of painkillers or surgery, we created a regeneration plan: physical therapy, PRP injections for his knee, low-impact cardio in the pool and on the bike, resistance training, and an anti-inflammatory diet. Six months later, Mark was 20 pounds lighter, stronger, and pain-free enough to join a pickup basketball game with his son. He felt like an athlete again—not chasing college glory, but enjoying life fully and actively.

Dana, 47, an ex-marathoner turned mom, felt unrecognizable from her athletic past—winded on stairs, stiff from desk work, and out of shape. Tests confirmed low muscle mass, slow metabolism, and below-average VO_2 max. We reignited her inner athlete with 30-minute functional strength sessions, low-impact cardio, and improved protein intake. Hormone and vitamin. support rounded out her plan. Within four months, Dana dropped body fat, regained muscle, and rebuilt her confidence. By 48, she even signed up for a half-marathon charity run—not to set records, but to prove to herself she still could.

Leon, 60, a Masters track athlete, refused to give up sprinting despite slower recovery and nagging injuries. Our testing revealed low testosterone and growth hormone, plus micro-injuries in his tendons and cartilage. We started supervised hormone optimization, regenerative peptide therapy, improved warm-ups, added recovery routines, and dialed in nutrition with protein, collagen, and creatine. The next season, Leon ran close to his times from a decade earlier, injury-free and energized. He says 60 now feels like 40, and he's proof that smart, guided science can keep athletes competitive well into later decades.

Just One Story

If just **one** of these stories resonates with you. If just **one** story reminds you of your situation. If just **one** gives you hope that you, too, can experience a before-and-after transformation just like someone else, then reading this book will be worth the time it takes. You've already purchased it anyway, so might as well invest four to five hours over the coming days to read it all the way to the end. Along the way, you'll learn the *how* behind the *who*—that is, what specifically these individuals changed, why they changed it, and how you can, too. Let's make the rest of your life the best of your life.

CHAPTER 2
Renew Your Mission

Robert was a high-powered executive, a CFO, successful by every measure. But as he approached 60, a number kept echoing in his mind—his own father had died at 60. His grandfather hadn't lived much longer than that. And so Robert felt like he was walking toward the same family-owned cliffdrop. An expiration date had been stamped on his life before he was born. Pick a metaphor, any metaphor. None you could think of is probably too dramatic for Robert's mindset at the time. *Am I about to start living on borrowed time?*

That worry wasn't abstract. He had a wife and children. He had a company he had built and a team who relied on him. He thought about his father missing milestones, about the absence felt at births and graduations, and he didn't want that story to repeat. Legacy was on his mind. He couldn't shake it off. He didn't want to. He didn't have a choice.

Like so many people in his position, Robert went to his doctor. The basic panel came back; nothing looked terrible. His doctor told him he was fine and seemed normal. But Robert knew "fine" and "normal" weren't enough. His family history told him otherwise. His gut said no, too.

That's when Robert found Velocity. We looked deeper, across multiple vectors—imaging, laboratory, family history, genetics. And the picture was clear: Robert wasn't simply "fine" or "normal"—utterly misleading and downright dismissive comments from a healthcare provider. No, Robert was at risk, and the risk was very not-fine and surely not-normal.

For Robert, the turning point wasn't a single test result. It was the convergence of everything. His family history. His own numbers. Like the calcium build-up and soft unstable plaques that we saw on advanced coronary testing. Everything pointed the same direction—to the cliff. Everything had to change. It was no longer about "staying fine" by someone else's definition. Robert realized he had to do whatever it took to ensure he wouldn't share the same fate as his father—so he could age gracefully and strongly into the grandfather his own children missed out on.

When I talked through all of this with Robert, what came up again and again was one special word: **legacy**. Robert had already achieved what many dream of; he'd built an amazing company and earned success by every external measure. But now he was thinking more existentially. *Is this all there is? That I just make a bunch of money, then one day drop dead?*

Every time he talked about his kids, his eyes lit up. His preteens were his "why," his reason for getting up and going to work. When he wavered or doubted himself, when the changes felt hard, we would bring him back to that moment of clarity: his kids. The life he wanted to share with them as they grew up and started their own families. The habits he wanted them to inherit. The father he wanted to be. One who would be present for them, even decades from then onwards. Then there was his wife. And all the promises they'd made each other when they were young, in love, and broke. All the travel they would do. The holidays with grandbabies. The camper or summer cottage or backyard in-ground pool or all of them. More than presents mattered was presence. The two of them and just the two of them, all these years later.

None of this would be Robert's if the status quo stayed put. And so Robert's mission renewed. His numbers didn't lie, and neither did he. He was in it for his family, his legacy, and the mark he would leave on the world by choosing to outlive his destiny. Robert was going to win.

• • • •

Why do humans get a long middle-life period? Other animals don't. Many mammals spend their prime years reproducing (or competing to reproduce), then skip to the not-so-golden years where their fate is as cruel as mother nature's worst storms. I'm reminded of a viral clip showing an older lion outcast by other, fitter males—the alpha of the pride, ousted to die alone on the savannah. I don't recall any mention of the ex-king's age; he looked young and strong enough to me. But that's how it goes in much of the animal kingdom; you fight, father, and fade. That's the way it is for most species.

Not us.

The Purpose of a Fiftysomething

Humans are different. Our lifespans include a broad later span where we are no longer at peak fertility or peak sprint speed, yet we keep living, leading, deciding, and teaching. Now, this is no evolutionary glitch; it's by design. There aren't many like us. But there are a notable few. I'll explain.

Consider social mammals that survive through harsh seasons. Like elephant herds that gather around matriarchs who remember all the old water holes; according to JT Safaris, which provides its patrons opportunities to view local wildlife:

> In the world of Loxodonta africana, the African elephant, the matriarch is the core of the family unit, holding a role that is defined by more than size or strength; it is her cognitive ability and memory that sustain the herd. Researchers often highlight the extensive neural networks within the elephant's temporal lobes, responsible for their astonishing memory. This highly developed area allows the matriarch to recall distant locations of water and forage, even across years and shifts in the landscape—a trait particularly vital during prolonged droughts.[2]

And this sort of mentoring behavior in elephants is scientifically supported as well. According to a 2011 paper in *Proceedings of the Royal Society B: Biological Sciences:*

> . . . [A]ge affects the ability of matriarchs to make ecologically relevant decisions in a domain critical to survival—the assessment of predatory threat. While groups consistently adjust their defensive behaviour to the greater threat of three roaring lions versus one, families with younger matriarchs typically under-react to roars from male lions despite the severe danger they represent. Sensitivity to this key threat increases with matriarch age and is greatest for the oldest matriarchs, who are likely to have accumulated the most experience. Our study provides the first empirical evidence that individuals within a social group may derive significant benefits from the influence of an older leader because of their enhanced ability to make crucial decisions about predatory threat, generating important insights into selection for longevity in cognitively advanced social mammals.[3]

Likewise, orca pods follow "menopausal" females who know migration routes in lean years. According to a March 2015 study in the journal *Current Biology:*

> Classic life-history theory predicts that

menopause should not occur because there should be no selection for survival after the cessation of reproduction. Yet, human females routinely live 30 years after they have stopped reproducing. Only two other species—killer whales (Orcinus orca) and short-finned pilot whales (Globicephala macrorhynchus)—have comparable postreproductive lifespans . . . One hypothesis is that postreproductive females act as repositories of ecological knowledge and thereby buffer kin against environmental hardships . . . We show three key results. First, postreproductively aged females lead groups during collective movement in salmon foraging grounds. Second, leadership by postreproductively aged females is especially prominent in difficult years when salmon abundance is low. This finding is critical because salmon abundance drives both mortality and reproductive success in resident killer whales. Third, females are more likely to lead their sons than they are to lead their daughters, supporting predictions of recent models of the evolution of menopause based on kinship dynamics. Our results show that postreproductive females may boost the fitness of kin through the transfer of ecological knowledge. The value gained from the wisdom of elders can help explain why female resident killer whales and humans continue to live long after they have stopped reproducing.[4]

Also, wolves thrive when older animals enforce order and transmit hunting patterns. From the wildlife conservation nonprofit *Living with Wolves*:

> Wolves play together into old age, they raise their young as a group, and they care for injured companions. When they lose a pack mate, there is evidence that they suffer and mourn that loss. When we look at wolves, we are looking at tribes—extended families, each with its own homeland, history, knowledge, and indeed, culture.
>
> Wolves communicate, collaborate and share knowledge across generations. The older wolves, as more experienced hunters, share hunting strategies and techniques with younger wolves, passing down knowledge from one generation to the next, maintaining a culture unique to that pack.[5]

The lesson repeats. When a group's survival depends on knowledge and coordination, the older ones are not extras. Not dead weight. No . . . they are guides. Stabilizers. Saviors even.

For tens of millennia, we humans repurposed that pattern and multiplied it. We are the knowledge-storing and -transmitting creature. We protect what we've learned—often the hardest way—in language, in ritual, in stories, in muscle memory, and in the silent habits of how a household runs and how a community eats, worships, farms, trades, fights, and reconciles. You get it now. The middle decades—your fifties and sixties—exist at the hinge between youthful force of nature and elder protector of your people. You can still *do*; you must also now *teach*. Biologically and anthropologically speaking, nature does not expect you to outwork the twenty-year-old. But you *are* expected to show them how not to waste effort, how to focus effort, and when to stop.

Anthropologists have long described something called the "grandmother effect." It's where families and bands with healthy older adults raise more surviving children because elders supply food, childcare, and knowledge that reduce risk. That same dynamic shows up in modern life. The "food" is not merely calories, but also perspective. It's the story a teenager hears at the right moment that steers them away from a bad choice. It's the calm correction in a tense meeting that prevents a costly mistake. It's the habit you model at home—going for an evening walk, cooking real food, turning off the phone—that becomes the next generation's normal. Consider the example of former First Lady Michelle Obama:

> ... Michelle Obama probably couldn't have been as good a mother as she's been during her tenure as First Lady if her own mother, Marian Robinson, hadn't decided to relocate to the White House in 2009 so she could, as she put it, "get to be Grandma" and help her

granddaughters "grow up before my eyes." Nor could many other young mothers, whose mothers or mothers-in-law are willing to put in the time to do some serious babysitting, manage to do as good a job as they do juggling the needs of their children while focusing, at least some of the time, on their careers.[6]

And observe how in earlier times, grandmothers played a far more noticeable role in childrearing due to women having children at younger ages. From the same article as above:

A generation ago, when the average age at first birth for a new mother was 25, it was typical for people to become grandparents in their early 50s, when they were still relatively young, relatively energetic, and relatively able to take over when new parents were at the end of their rope . . . Grandma and Grandpa continued to have a role in the grandchildren's lives as the children grew up: the kids graduated from high school, and the grandparents were in their early 70s; graduated from college, and the grandparents were in their mid-70s; married, and the grandparents were in their early 80s and probably still sufficiently agile to get to the wedding.[7]

That's a long time to be productive while postreproductive. And that seems to be nature's design. As you might expect, there is evidence pointing to the idea that a long post-fertility period is a distinctive human adaptation.[8]

And now the deeper purpose of midlife is revealed— **to transmit the wisdom that keeps others alive and well**.

If you only hear midlife as a countdown to decline, you miss the job description baked into your biology. Middle years are like a baton pass. You are receiving the full weight of what came before, and you are responsible for handing forward something better.

This is what we are building towards. Your health in your fifties and beyond is different from health at all other ages. In your twenties and maybe thirties, physical health was there for looking good and sharp, probably staying athletic as well. By your forties, health is about sustenance—to keep going. By now, it's not just everything . . . it's all there is. You now have a prehistoric job to live long and well enough to show the way. A strong body and clear mind are not for vanity. They're resources that make you uniquely valuable as a human being.

In case you needed any additional convincing, simply consider the catastrophe when there was no steady soul in the room. A business gets derailed by impulsive decisions. A family fracture deepens because no one has the energy to listen. A preventable medical crisis becomes a tragedy because no one paid attention to quiet warnings. Midlife gives you the chance to be the person who pays attention, slows impulsive moves, and has the bandwidth (and depth) to notice what matters. That's Robert's story. What jolted him wasn't bloodwork. It was that expiration date. The worry that he was going to miss so much. The realization even. He started asking the questions that undergird this chapter: W*ho needs me? What do they need from me? Am I physically and mentally capable of giving it to them for the next twenty years? If not, what must change now?*

A body that **sleeps** consistently can listen and decide. A brain **fed** by stable blood sugar and supported by **muscle** does not fall apart at the first sign of stress. **Hormones** in healthy ranges change how you interpret risk, how you regulate emotion, and how you lead. When you improve those levers, you become the adult everyone assumes you already are. You develop better judgment. Get more patience. A longer fuse. A steady capacity to carry weight without dropping it. It's incredible.

But biology will **not** do all this for you automatically. Nature gives you the assignment; you must accept it. Most people don't. They arrive at the middle and think the job is to hang on. And so the decline begins. Many assume their best years are behind them; the body believes it. Long meetings, travel, stress, sleep debt, social drinking, easy calories, no movement. It all adds up; subtraction by addition. Ironic, isn't it? Less quality of life now, less life later. This is not what I want for you. Midlife is the most leveraged period of your life. I want you to use it.

Please don't wait for a scare to discover this. Steal Robert's shortcut and make it yours. Time isn't guaranteed. What his family needs most is him, present and steady.

So I encourage you: Decide that the job of midlife is to carry people into their future with more strength than you were given. Then build the health that lets you do it. And so this is the biological and anthropological purpose of your fifties—to become the person others can lean on without falling yourself. It is an **honor**; it is also your **duty**.

An Honor and a Duty

Like certain animal species, different human cultures tell a story about the middle years. The specifics vary; the assignment does not. At midlife, you are called to responsibility that is larger than your personal ambition. You are asked to hold a role—sometimes formal, often invisible—that protects others, transmits values, and steadies the next generation.

In Classical India

In the Indian tradition, life is mapped as a progression of *ashramas*: student, householder, forest-dweller, renunciate. According to the Hindu American Foundation, the *ashramas* work like so:

> *Brahmacharya* is the first stage of life. It is the student stage of life, preparing for success in later stages of life . . . The second stage is called *Grihastha* . . . [I]t follows what most people do naturally after leaving

school: Maintaining a home, having a family .
. *Vanaprashta* is the third stage . . . In ancient
times, once reaching this stage people would
start detaching themselves from family life
and the pursuit of material ends by moving to
the forest time to devote more of their time to
spiritual practice, living among other seekers
of solace, knowledge, peace, and freedom . . .
The fourth stage is *Sannyasa,* renunciation . .
. A *sannyasin* (women renunciates are called
sannyasini) lives a very simple life, subsisting
on a minimum of material possessions and
devoting themselves to nonviolence.[9]

The labels are poetic, but the message is practical.
You study and train. Then you build a household
and contribute. After that, you release your grip on
accumulation and redirect attention to meaning. Finally,
you devote yourself to what lasts. Midlife is the liminal
space between householder and forest-dweller. You still
lead and provide; you also start shaping how your people
will live when you are not there.

In the Gita, Arjuna stands on a battlefield, paralyzed
by doubt. He does not want the role he has been given.
He would prefer peace without conflict. Krishna instructs
him to act according to *dharma*, not preference.[10] Do
the work that is yours to do. The lesson travels cleanly
into a boardroom, a kitchen, a clinic. Often at midlife
you are the only person in the room who can do the hard
thing without making it worse. You speak when others
are afraid to, and you stay quiet when talking would only

satisfy your ego. You bear the weight of hard decisions so younger shoulders don't have to.

This is duty.

In Ancient Rome (And Greece)

A world away, Roman writers gave midlife a slightly different frame. They obsessed less over stages and more over virtues. *Gravitas, constantia, humanitas.* In *De Senectute* Cicero reminds his readers that old age is not a thief, if properly prepared for; no, it is a crown of capacities that do not fade—judgment, counsel, dignity.[11] That said, Greco-Roman philosophers also had specific virtues for specific ages and stages. For example, in adulthood, *arete* (ἀρετή) is a core concept meaning excellence, virtue, and the fulfillment of potential.

Now, back to the virtues, the classical Roman model places a high bar on behavior. A leader in the middle years must be stable enough to absorb shocks and humble enough to take advice. They must serve the republic, not the self. Over time, this becomes honor—the earned authority that comes from doing what is right when no one can force you.

In Royal China

Back in the East—the Far East this time—Confucian thought has cast the assignment of middle age as relational. The elder has obligations up and down the family tree—to honor those who came before, to teach those who come after, and to conduct themselves with propriety so the social fabric holds. The key word is *ren*: humaneness.[12] Duty cannot be divorced from kindness. You see, authority isn't license to dominate or otherwise boss people around, i.e., "I'm older than you, so I'm in charge here." No; it is a responsibility to relieve burdens. In that world, a middle-aged adult who does not restrain impulses or cultivate virtue is failing both the ancestors and the descendants—and the culture and its people at large.

In Middle-Ages Japan

A short way across the sea, the Japanese had added a word that neatly bridges duty and joy: *ikigai*. It is the reason you get up in the morning—the place where what you love, what you're good at, what the world needs, and what you can be paid for overlap.[13]

In Native Americans

Native American elders are basically libraries. They keep the songs, the maps, the medicine, and the stories of what went wrong last time. And so honor is bestowed upon them not because of status but service. If you hoard knowledge—or worse, dismiss it all together—you lose standing. If you share it, you rise.

Among Plains Indians, for example, older women kept the history of the tribe:

> The maturing Plains Indian women devoted
> themselves to daily prayer with the same

reverent spirituality they had practiced as younger women. The end of childbearing years marked an important passage for women into a realm of respect and distinction . . .The women elders instilled the ancient traditions, lore, and values of their people to their grandchildren. They helped their granddaughters master the traditional skills and crafts of their tribe. The maturing Plains Indian women completed the circle of their lives by guiding new generations in the path of their ancestors.[14]

Likewise, Navajo elder women have played a similar role:

Navajo grandmothers are revered not only for their roles as matriarchs but also for their wisdom, guidance, and nurturing qualities. They take on the responsibility of passing down cultural knowledge, teaching traditional skills, and instilling moral values in their grandchildren.[15]

Naturally, the older men aren't sitting around doing nothing either. Among the Lakota Sioux, older men held many important roles:

In traditional Lakota community life, fraternal societies, called *akicitas*, are significant within the life of the group. During the era of the buffalo when Lakota society was highly mobile, fraternal societies helped young men develop leadership skills by assigning them roles in maintaining orderly camp movements. Membership was by invitation only and restricted to the most promising young men. Another kind of fraternity, the *nacas,* was composed of older men with proven abilities.[16]

Also, Sioux grandparents in general were often entrusted with the primary responsibility for caring for small children and infants and assisting with household tasks.[17] Indeed, the role of lore-keeper is common for the elderly is across numerous Native American tribes:

> In many traditional Indian societies, old age brought respect and leadership. It was understood that the experience and knowledge of elders was a resource that could be drawn upon as a tribe made decisions for the future . . . "All of our elders, because of their life experiences, their wisdom, are very valuable to us," said Clarence Woodcock, director of the Salish Cultural Center on the Flathead Reservation. "The gifts they have been given—their knowledge of our culture, traditions, our general lifeways—are valuable and because of that we honor them."[18]

The Natives of old did not treat elderhood like a second childhood but as a profound responsibility to those who come after them (but to be fair to modern seniors, they do see their grandchildren two to four times per month.)[19]

In The Modern First World

Your fifties are the moment to clarify and live without apology. What else are you going to do with this period and what comes after? Italian wine-tasting? French Riviera sightseeing? Monthlong cruises around Antarctica?

Unfortunately, too many older people in our 21st-century world do exactly that. Let's look at some numbers.

A Late-Adulthood Revival of Adolescence

The average age of guests on river cruises is now 55 years old, down from 66 in 2019.[20] Younger and younger, leisure spending is going up and up. Gen X accounts for most luxury purchases, followed by older Millennials.[21] Baby Boomers make up the largest share of new home buyers at 42 percent.[22]

And most importantly for this point, only 22 percent of Boomers plan to leave an inheritance.[23] This takes on particular salience, since as of this writing economic times are difficult and high home prices have put property ownership out of reach for a lot of young people. To make matters worse, those high home prices. It is at the heart of much of the young's grumbling about the older generations. A 2024 article in the *New York Post* describes a movement called "spending your kids' inheritance" (SKI), in which parents seek to spend out their money so that their children are left with nothing.[24]

This obvious selfishness is frequently framed as a way for elderly people to help their adult sons and daughters by teaching them the value of hard work and earning their own keep, as well as showing them that they can't expect something for nothing. A common fear is that inheritors will become spoiled and waste the money, so expecting financial help even in uncertain economic times is treated as a grown-up version of asking for a pony.

Financial advising company *Become* justifies SKI with the following:

1. Life Is Way Too Short to Delay Having Fun, the Best Years Often Come Early in Retirement

2. A Decent Slice of Inheritances Are Squandered

3. Experiences Beat "stuff" For Lasting Happiness

4. Too Much of an Inheritance Can Dilute the Ethics You Most Value

5. Estates Can Be Slow, Costly, and Sometimes Messy[25]

TV personality Simon Cowell, the man who famously ripped into poor performers during the audition segments of *American Idol,* has said that he does not plan to leave any of his fortune to his children. According to him, "College will be paid for, and then you're on your own."[26]

While Cowell isn't completely leaving his kids hanging, it's telling that he believes leaving them an inheritance would harm them. And to be fair, it's not as if parents who deny their children an inheritance did nothing for those children as they grew up. I am not alleging neglect on their part, or a failure to teach them appropriate values.

The issue here is how we've recontextualized old age. Our modern culture turns holidays and getaways into must-haves—the thing we're supposed to do all the time once we're aged and "deserve it." It's an odd sort of adolescent pleasure-seeking, isn't it?

Dare I say that all of the above is unnatural behavior from our elders? I do dare. Because it is. Sadly, the modern default for most of us as we age is not the *ashramas, ren, arete,* or anything like that. Imagine in North America an old Native chief. Can you imagine the elders of the tribe waving away all the younger folks and going off to enjoy their latter years, leaving nothing for their children or grandchildren? It's absurd in this context.

The True Purpose of Midlife

Across all traditions the world over, one truth is constant down through the generations—**midlife belongs to contribution**. That's where the meaning is. It's the balance between drudgery and living for another and nostalgia and living for yourself—it's the best of both worlds. That's why we need you to be as healthy as possible for as long as possible. Because duty without capacity breeds resentment. Honor without energy will become senior-citizen cosplay. If you are going to accept your next social role, you need stamina. That means telling yourself the truth about your body and its status quo.

That's how you take your power back from Father Time, so you can serve humanity like Mother Nature intended. That's what Robert did. He found his mission, his *why*. Let's secure yours now.

The Five *Why's* for Your Midlife Mission

Simon Sinek's concept of the Five *Why's* is a simple tool to uncover the deepest reason behind a goal or a problem. From his early viral TED Talk, dating way, way back to ancient internet history in 2010 (but ultimately originating from the process improvement of the Toyota automobile company):

> Why is it that Martin Luther King led the Civil Rights Movement? He wasn't the only man who suffered in pre-civil rights America, and he certainly wasn't the only great orator of the day.
>
> Why him?
>
> And why is it that the Wright brothers were able to figure out controlled, powered man flight when there were certainly other teams who were better qualified, better funded --

and they didn't achieve powered man flight, and the Wright brothers beat them to it.

There's something else at play here . . . [V] ery, very few people or organizations know why they do what they do. And by "why" I don't mean ""to make a profit." That's a result. It's always a result.

By "why," I mean: What's your purpose? What's your cause? What's your belief? Why does your organization exist? Why do you get out of bed in the morning? And why should anyone care?

As a result, the way we think, we act, the way we communicate is from the outside in, it's obvious. We go from the clearest thing to the fuzziest thing.

But the inspired leaders and the inspired organizations—regardless of their size, regardless of their industry—all think, act and communicate from the inside out.[27]

This is no mere self-help hucksterism on Sinek's part. From a 2014 paper in *Psychological Science:*

Having a purpose in life has been nominated consistently as an indicator of healthy aging for several reasons including its potential for reducing mortality risk . . . [P]urposeful individuals lived longer than their counterparts during the 14 years after assessment, even when controlling for other markers of psychological and affective well-being. Moreover, these longevity benefits do not appear to be conditional on either the participants' age, how long they lived, or whether they had retired from the workforce. In other words, having a purpose appears to widely buffer against mortality risk across the adult years.[28]

So, how do you run this exercise? You start with a statement (goal or obstacle), then ask "Why?" five times. Each answer becomes the next prompt. By the fifth why, you're usually staring at the real truth, the one with enough emotional mass to attract action.

Here's a little more on how to do the exercise:

- Write the first statement exactly as it sits in your head.

- Ask "Why?" and answer in one or two honest sentences. No polishing.

- Use the previous answer as the next prompt. Ask "Why?" again. Repeat five times.

- If you get stuck, ask, "What would make this matter so much that I'd do it even when I'm busy or tired?"

- When an answer makes you feel something—a lump in the throat, a pull in the gut—you've hit the root.

Pro tip: Do this for multiple domains. You're building mission density. The more overlapping, emotionally real *why's* you have, the steadier your consistency will be.

Let's form some *"Why* Trees" so you'll know how to make yours, too.

Why Tree 1: "Why do you want to get healthy?"

Statement: I want to get healthy.

- *Why* #1: Why do you want to get healthy?
  Answer: Because I'm tired of waking up drained and dragging through the day.

- *Why* #2: Why does waking up drained matter?
  Answer: Because it makes me impatient with my family and sloppy at work; I'm not the person I want to be in either place.

- *Why* #3: Why does being that person matter to you?
  Answer: Because my kids and my team look to me for stability, and lately I'm the one wobbling.

- *Why* #4: Why is being their stability so important?
  Answer: Because I grew up without it. My father was gone before 60, and everything felt precarious after that.

- *Why* #5: Why do you need to break that pattern now?
  Answer: Because I refuse to hand my children that same insecurity. Getting healthy is how I become the steady center our family can count on.

Root you can use: *Get healthy so my family never has to feel the instability I felt. I will be the steady center.*
Other real-world root variations readers might land on:

- *So I can be fully present, not half-awake and irritable.*

- *So I can stop numbing out with food, alcohol, or screens and actually show up for my life.*

- *So I can earn back self-respect one decision at a time.*

Why Tree 2: "Why do you want to leave a legacy?"

Statement: I want to leave a legacy.

- *Why* #1: Why do you want to leave a legacy?
Answer: Because I want my life to add up to more than a résumé and a balance sheet.

- *Why* #2: Why does "more than a résumé and a balance sheet" matter?
Answer: Because I've hit goals before and felt empty the next day. It fades fast.

- *Why* #3: Why do those wins feel empty for you?
Answer: Because they don't outlive me. Values and example do. Money, titles, buildings—they're temporary.

- *Why* #4: Why is passing down values and example urgent now?

Answer: Because my kids and the people I lead are watching how I handle midlife. If I drift, they learn drifting. If I choose purpose, they learn purpose.

- *Why #5*: Why is modeling purpose the legacy you want?
Answer: Because the loudest thing I can leave behind is who I became when it was hardest. I want them to inherit that story.

Root you can use: *Leave a legacy of example, not just assets. The story I live now is what my family and team will carry.*

Other real-world root variations:

- *To honor the sacrifices my parents made by building something that lasts beyond me.*

- *To give my children a ladder of habits and principles, not just a check.*

- *To shift our family story from surviving to thriving.*

Why Tree 3: "Why is it important to you to live a long time?"

Statement: It's important to me to live a long time.

- *Why #1*: Why is living a long time important?
Answer: Because I want to see my kids become who they're meant to be—and maybe meet my grandkids.

- *Why #2*: Why do those future moments matter

so much?
Answer: Because they're the point. Work is meaningful, but family milestones are the irreplaceable moments.

- *Why* #3: Why do you believe family moments outrank professional milestones?
Answer: Because when I picture the end of my life, I don't regret missed meetings. I regret missed time with people I love.

- *Why* #4: Why is that vision at the end pushing you now?
Answer: Because I've watched people run out the clock earlier than they had to. It's needless loss when we ignore preventable risks.

- *Why* #5: Why does preventing that loss feel like a personal mandate?
Answer: Because I can control many of the risks. Choosing health adds years, and more importantly, adds good days to those years.

Root you can use: *Live long to stack irreplaceable moments with the people I love. Add good days, not just years.*

Other real-world root variations:

- *To finish the work only I can do and hand it off well.*

- *To see the next tech revolutions through with clarity and contribute, not spectate.*

- *To grow old with my partner in strength and joy, not decline.*

Why Tree 4: "Why do you want to stay active into your latter years?"

Statement: I want to stay active into my latter years.

- *Why* #1: Why do you want to stay active later in life?

  Answer: Because I want to travel, hike, and play with future grandkids without sitting it out.

- *Why* #2: Why is participating, not spectating, important to you?

  Answer: Because activity is freedom. Watching from the bench feels like missing my own life.

- *Why* #3: Why does "freedom" show up as the key word?

  Answer: Because I've seen what losing mobility looks like. It shrinks your world to a chair, a room, a schedule someone else controls.

- *Why* #4: Why does avoiding that shrinkage matter beyond comfort?

  Answer: Because purpose needs a body that can carry it. If I can move, I can contribute.

- *Why* #5: Why is contributing in your later years central to your identity?

  Answer: Because my value isn't over at 60. Activity keeps me useful, engaged, and alive to my mission.

Root you can use: *Stay active to stay free and useful.*

Mobility is how I keep contributing.

Other real-world root variations:

- *So I can say yes to adventures instead of apologizing for my limitations.*

- *So movement stays a joy, not a chore or a risk.*

- *So my latter years expand my world, not shrink it.*

Why Tree 5: "Why do you want to be able to live independently as you age?"

Statement: I want to live independently as I age.

- *Why* #1: Why do you want independence later in life?

  Answer: Because I don't want to be a burden on my kids.

- *Why* #2: Why does "not being a burden" matter deeply?

  Answer: Because I watched a parent lose independence, and it pulled the whole family under stress we weren't ready for.

- *Why* #3: Why did that experience mark you?

  Answer: Because we lost time with them to logistics and crisis. The relationship became tasks, not connection.

- *Why* #4: Why is preserving connection over tasks your priority?

  Answer: Because love is the point, not caretaking paperwork. Independence protects the relationships I care about.

- *Why* #5: Why is protecting those relationships worth changing your habits now?
  Answer: Because every choice I make today either preserves future dignity and closeness or erodes it. I want dignity and closeness.

Root you can use: *Protect dignity and connection. Stay independent so our time is love, not logistics.*
Other real-world root variations:

- *So my children can visit me for joy, not obligation.*

- *So I choose where I live and how I spend my days, not an intake form.*

- *So I can keep giving, not only receiving.*

May you find your *why*. And know that it's never too late to do so.

A final lesson is for anyone in midlife who thinks they are behind. You are not. You are right on time . . . if you start now, if not sooner. Biology responds to clear direction. Labs can improve in weeks. Strength returns. Sleep stabilizes. Mood evens out. The harder thing is not the protocol; it is keeping your reason visible. That is the work that keeps all the other work doable.

Robert will close this chapter because his story began it. He stopped seeing himself as a man walking toward a cliff and started living as a father and leader building a longer road. That is the win in the clinic that matters to me most. When someone stops fearing their life and starts using it, starts living it.

Robert's Mission, Continued

Throughout his time with us, Robert's mission became his anchor. Whenever life got busy, whenever he slipped on his workouts or stopped logging his meals, we would bring him back to the words he himself had spoken early on. His why. His kids. His family. His legacy.

There wasn't a smoking gun or a dramatic movie moment. For Robert, the vision of a future he wouldn't earn if he didn't fight for it . . . that carried him through the difficult stretches.

When he achieved milestones—like reaching his target body fat percentage—we sent him a congratulations letter that mentioned his family. He shared it with his wife and children. It meant the world to him because it was more than proof of health achievement; it showed his mission was alive and real. And he was in the process of accomplishing it. All of it.

See, Robert's renewed mission wasn't (just) about avoiding an untimely and sudden death. He had a duty to his progeny; he simply *decided* he would succeed where his own ancestors failed. When the biggest questions of life are answered, when you know what you're living for, health becomes fuel. It becomes who you are. This is just what you do. And this new self-knowledge grants you an inner peace unlike any other—one that also happens to quiet the restless mind and carry you into the night with a calm, unshakeable resolve.

CHAPTER 3
Rejuvenate with Sleep

"You need to lose weight. You probably need to get your hormones checked, too."

That's what Laura kept hearing. But the well-meaning advice from friends, co-workers, and even doctors who gave her the usual checklist of midlife fixes felt . . . *mean*. Unrealistic at best, cruel at worst.

As you read in Chapter 1, Laura's reality at age 50 was, effectively, to try to live three lives at once. There's more to her story than I've shared, so much more that it will make sense why her story opens this chapter.

By day, Laura was a professional with a steady nine-to-five job. She clocked in, kept things running, and got the bills paid. By evening, she was Mom chasing around two teenagers—a boy and a girl—with two sets of adolescent anxiety to allay. And, of course, two sets of activities to take them to. And also by night—the same night, every night—Laura was a caregiver for her father, whose health had declined so much so fast that she'd basically become an STNA for him at the nearby nursing home. Between and among all of this, there just wasn't a spare minute that belonged to Laura. How, exactly, is a woman like this going to just lose weight? Just monitor and adjust as needed her hormonal levels? Just start taking care of herself when everyone around her needs her? Just cruel.

Now, from the outside, it probably looked to naïve family and friends like Laura was managing OK enough—job, kids, caregiving. In reality, she was burnt to the embers. Most nights followed the same exhausting script. She'd leave work, stop in to sit with her dad and advocate for him with the staff, head home, cook (or heat up a package of) dinner, help her teens with whatever needed doing, and finally—finally—collapse onto the living room couch around 11:00 to 11:30 p.m. The house was quiet; all were asleep. This was her one shot at freedom and self-care every day.

And how do you suppose she'd spend it? Well, I can't blame her. Like so many others in her situation, Laura would "unwine" with a glass (or two or three) of mid-market merlot. She scrolled Facebook and TikTok. She'd stream a few episodes of whatever popcorn show the Netflix algorithm suggested. Sometimes she raided the pantry for salty snacks or late-night sweets. All this added up—her little rebellion against the nonstop demands of everyone.

But what Laura called self-care was, in fact, self-sabotage. The alcohol helped her fall asleep faster but prevented her body from dropping into deep, restorative sleep. The blue light from her screens tricked her brain into thinking it was still daytime. The ultra-processed foods she reached for kept her blood sugar wild; she'd jolt awake at 2:00 a.m. or toss and turn till dawn.

By the time she finally crawled into bed around 1:15 a.m. each night, Laura was a shell of herself. Stress hormones reverberated within. To-do lists bounced off each wall of her mind. And every morning, she woke up more exhausted than she felt when collapsing on the covers.

The poor-sleep debt had to be paid. And so it had been. Laura had gained twenty pounds over the past few years. Her joints ached constantly. She felt inflamed, foggy, irritable. She relied on caffeine to get through the day, then the alcohol to wind down at night. She was locked in an escapeless loop. Her annual labs showed that she was edging toward diabetes, with her hemoglobin A1C hovering at 6.2 percent. Her doctor shrugged and said, "We'll keep an eye on it."

Remind you of Robert? Me too. Of course, "keeping an eye on it" wasn't working for anyone. Laura was so far beyond tired at this point. Empty, depleted, gone.

When she finally came to Velocity Health from a referral, she brought the same complaints so many midlife patients bring, like weight gain, fatigue, mood swings, and brain fog. She expected to hear the same prescriptions she'd heard before about diet and exercise and maybe hormone therapy. Instead, we asked her a different question during intake.

"Can you tell us about your sleep?"

That's when everything finally made sense to her. Laura admitted she hadn't slept through the night in years. She laughed with bitter sarcasm when asked if she woke up feeling rested.

"Rested? I don't even remember what that feels

like," she said.

We ran a Dutch test, which measures cortisol throughout the day. A healthy curve rises in the morning and gently falls toward bedtime, signaling the body to power down. Laura's curve was inverted—her stress hormone spiked early, stayed high all day, but barely dropped at night. She was essentially living in a twenty-four-seven fight-or-flight state.

Laura just needed to sleep. Some real, restorative, deep sleep. So that's where we started—with the fundamentals of sleep hygiene. At our suggestion, Laura shut down screens an hour before bed. She also swapped the wine for herbal tea. She journaled for ten minutes each night to dump her racing thoughts onto paper, sometimes her laptop (with blue light-blocking glasses). We also added a gentle magnesium supplement to help her relax going into sleep. And finally, her bedroom became a sanctuary—dark, cool, and screen-free.

This is where Laura's new story begins. With this book, it's where yours can, too.

Why Sleep First

Why must sleep be the first change you make? Because lack of sleep—or poor-quality sleep—makes everything else going wrong in your body far, far worse and far, far sooner, as Laura herself observed. It's unfortunately common to see someone with disrupted or inadequate sleep struggle across every other area of health. Regulate sleep, and suddenly it becomes easier to make better choices with food, movement, stress, and relationships.

Leave sleep unchecked, and all those areas spiral.

During sleep, your body does its deepest repair work, and your brain flushes out toxins. Hormones rebalance, memories consolidate, and cognition sharpens. Quality sleep lowers the risks of heart disease, obesity, diabetes, depression, and dementia. Screw this up, and so becomes everything else.

But how important is sleep to the body? It goes beyond recovering from tiredness. Good sleep also:

- **Heals and repairs your heart and blood vessels.**

- **Helps support a healthy balance of the hormones that make you feel hungry (ghrelin) or full (leptin):** When you don't get enough sleep, your level of ghrelin goes up and your level of leptin goes down. This makes you feel hungrier than when you're well-rested.

- **Affects how your body reacts to insulin:** Insulin is the hormone that controls your blood glucose (sugar) level. Sleep deficiency results in a higher-than-normal blood sugar level, which may raise your risk of diabetes.

- **Supports healthy growth and development:** Deep sleep triggers the body to release the hormone that promotes normal growth in children and teens. This hormone also boosts muscle mass and helps repair cells and tissues in children, teens, and adults. Sleep also plays a role in puberty and fertility.

- **Affects your body's ability to fight germs and sickness:** Ongoing sleep deficiency can change the way your body's natural defense against germs and sickness responds. For example, if you're sleep deficient, you may have trouble fighting common infections.

- **Decreases your risk of health problems, including heart disease, high blood pressure, obesity, and stroke.**[29]

Now, if "just get better sleep to get better everything else" were so easy, we all would do it, of course. More information does not mean more motivation. Sleep is one of the hardest habits to improve because it's tangled up with modern life. So much of what we do happens late at night because that's all the time left. It's cramming for a test, and there's one every day. We try finishing work, binge-watching shows, scrolling through feeds, grabbing food, catching up on emails, even doing household chores—even outdoor ones! I have some neighbors you wouldn't believe. You probably do, too. The sleep problem is ubiquitous. According to the Centers for Disease Control:

> A growing number of American workers are not getting enough sleep. Research shows an increase from 24% in the 1980s to 30% in the 2000s in the percentage of American civilian workers reporting 6 or fewer hours of sleep per day—a level considered by sleep experts to be too short . . . Work demands are one factor. The timing of a shift can

strain a worker's ability to get enough sleep. Working at night or during irregular hours goes against the human body's biology, which is hard-wired to sleep during the night and be awake and active during the day.[30]

If that doesn't describe the world of remote work, I don't know what does. The gig economy and entry-level jobs are also in play here as much as the laptop-worker and white-collar classes. A 2020 study in *SSM - Population Health* pins some blame on unpredictable service sector schedules:

> In the retail and food service sectors, work schedules change from day-to-day and week-to-week, often with little advance notice, posing a potential impediment to healthy sleep patterns . . . We find that the unstable and unpredictable schedules that are typical in the service sector are associated with poor sleep quality, difficulty falling asleep, waking during sleep, and waking up feeling tired . . . The strength of the associations between most types of unstable and unpredictable work schedules and sleep quality are stronger than those of having a pre-school aged child or working a regular night shift.[31]

Even physicians like me who should know better aren't immune to late-night work ethic temptation (and frankly, to petty distractions also).One of the densest usage periods where healthcare practitioners access and annotate electronic health records (EHR) is late evening. According to the *Annals of Family Medicine,* "Primary care physicians spend more than one-half of their workday, nearly 6 hours, interacting with the EHR during and after clinic hours."[32] We're scrambling to finish notes at home after shifts; the "and" in that sentence is no small afterthought.

Now, since we know what we're supposed to do with regards to sleep, why don't we just do it? Actually, no . . . that's not quite correct. "Just get better sleep" is the kind of eye-rolling non-advice everyone hates. What are we *actually* supposed to do so that better sleep is *actually* the natural outcome of our nights? That's the real question. Laura got quick tips like these to get her started:

- **Prioritize sleep as non-negotiable**. Aim for 7-8 hours of quality rest in a dark, cool room, with a consistent schedule and a wind-down routine.

- **Obey the 3-2-1 Rule**. Three hours before bed, stop eating. Two hours before bed, step away from screens. One hour before bed, cut off fluids so your bladder doesn't wake you.

- **Limit blue light**. Blue-light-blocking glasses aren't perfect, but they help. Better yet, replace screen time with something restorative—an evening walk, conversation with your spouse, journaling, and such.

- **Get evaluated**. Many people have

undiagnosed sleep conditions like sleep apnea. A sleep study can uncover hidden issues. Supplements like magnesium or in some cases peptides can help restore balance.

These are a helpful start. Even so, there's more you can do—much more. At Velocity Health, we teach what we call the **Sleep Symphony**. These are the ten factors that, when tuned together, create the conditions for the best sleep of your life for the rest of your life. Let's hear it.

The Sleep Symphony

Play each of these well, and you will hear absolutely . . . nothing. Because you will be asleep. The slightest noise won't rustle you. I would say you wouldn't believe it, but, again, you'll be asleep. Let's get you some rest. Here are ten "instruments" to play and one straightforward and practical method for you to start playing them today. Beginning with . . .

The Hormone Help

Melatonin is the body's timekeeper, originating from serotonin through the tryptophan-serotonin biosynthesis process in the pineal gland. The gut is also a major source of melatonin, producing much more than the pineal. When the intestinal barrier becomes permeable due to inflammation or dysbiosis, pathogens and endotoxins activate the immune system and induce cytokines like IL-1β, IL-6, IL-18, and interferon-γ. These cytokines stimulate IDO (indoleamine 2,3-dioxygenase), which diverts tryptophan away from melatonin synthesis and reduces levels. Without adequate serotonin, melatonin synthesis falters, especially in low-light environments.

A 2023 paper in *Cell and Molecular Neurobiology* points out that "Melatonin production and release peak during the dark hours and fall during the day in all species studied."[33] It also clarifies that melatonin is created at night with its peak concentration in the blood found around 3:00 to 4:00 a.m.[34] Given these times in which melatonin is generated and when it dissipates, melatonin is perfectly timed to match a normal sleep cycle.

There's more. Adenosine acts as the pressure valve for sleep, building throughout the day as ATP breaks down, then clearing during slow-wave sleep. From a May 2022 paper in the *Journal of Sleep Research:*

> Adenosine is a breakdown product of the depletion of ATP in the brain . . . After prolonged neuronal activity during wakefulness, ATP accumulates in the extracellular space and is degraded by 5'-EN to adenosine. Adenosine is thought to increase in the extracellular space in the course of prolonged waking, and has been proposed as a homeostatic accumulator of the need to sleep.[35]

Furthermore, in the same paper:

> In several regions of the brain, stimulation

of adenosine A_1 receptors depresses glutamate release, reducing the amplitude of postsynaptic currents . . . The accumulation of adenosine . . . may therefore reduce the activity of wake promoting areas and, in this way, disinhibit sleep promoting areas.[36]

But caffeine blocks adenosine receptors; this lowers sleep pressure and impairs clearance, leaving you groggy the next day. The paper explains this:

Caffeine is a potent adenosine receptor antagonist with roughly equally high affinity for both A_1 and A_{2A} receptors . . . [C]affeine promotes wakefulness primarily by blocking the A_{2A} subtype of adenosine receptors.[37]

It becomes clear that caffeine will harm your ability to sleep if taken close to bedtime.[38] And we can't forget cortisol. Cortisol peaks in the morning to promote alertness, then falls in the evening to allow sleep. According to a January 2021 paper in the *International Journal of Environmental Research and Public Health,* cortisol secretion peaks at 7 to 8 AM, and is at its lowest at 2 to 4 AM.[39] But this isn't a hard-and-fast rule; according to a 2022 paper in *Frontiers in Neuroscience,* cortisol peaks about an hour after waking up.[40]

Elevated cortisol at night—due to stress, circadian disruption, or blue light—suppresses melatonin and reduces deep and REM sleep. From a November 2020 paper published by the National Institutes of Health:

In normal individuals, wakefulness and stage 1 sleep (light sleep) accompany cortisol increases, while slow wave sleep or deep sleep is associated with declining plasma cortisol levels. In addition, in normals, induced sleep disruption (frequently repeated arousals) is associated with significant increases of plasma cortisol levels. Furthermore, mean 24-hour plasma cortisol levels are significantly higher in subjects with a shorter total sleep time than those with a longer total sleep time.[41]

Slow wave (deep) sleep is also called the N3 stage. It's when brain activity slows into high-amplitude, low-frequency waves, the body becomes hardest to wake, and (importantly for performance and long-term health) physiology shifts toward repair, restoration, and cellular housekeeping. The brain and body can rebalance energy allocation, which is more than simply "rest" but rather a coordinated shift that supports cellular renewal at the level of mitochondria.[42]

This sort of disruption even has a role to play in insomnia:

Insomnia, the most common sleep disorder, is associated with a 24hour increase of ACTH and cortisol secretion, consistent with a disorder of central nervous system hyperarousal.[43]

Also:

> ... [T]he 24-hour ACTH and cortisol plasma concentrations were significantly higher in insomniacs than matched normal controls. Within the 24-hour period, the greatest elevations were observed in the evening and first half of the night. Also, insomniacs with a high degree of objective sleep disturbance (% sleep time < 70) secreted a higher amount of cortisol, compared to those with a low degree of sleep disturbance.[44]

Bright light at night suppresses melatonin, too, with reductions of about 14 percent documented, though there wasn't a strong effect on sleep quality.[45]

Other hormones play supporting roles. DHEA buffers cortisol and stabilizes the stress response. Progesterone has natural sedative effects by enhancing GABA transmission, reducing sleep latency, and supporting consolidated non-REM sleep. What is GABA, you might wonder? That's the brain's off-switch. You don't want that not working.

One (More) Thing You Can Do Starting Now: Control your light exposure at night. Dim lights and cut screens in the last two hours before bed so melatonin can rise and cortisol can fall—which will over time help foster the hormonal conditions necessary for restorative sleep. Per a 2010 study in the *Journal of Clinical Endocrinology and Metabolism*:

Compared with dim light, exposure to room light before bedtime suppressed melatonin, resulting in a later melatonin onset in 99.0% of individuals and shortening melatonin duration by about 90 min. Also, exposure to room light during the usual hours of sleep suppressed melatonin by greater than 50% in most (85%) trials.[46]

There are few studies where the number "99.0%" occurs. Now you understand why sleep is the first of the Core Four.

Sleep-Timing It Right

When you go to sleep is as important as how long you sleep. Variability in sleep-wake cycles desynchronizes circadian rhythms—the body's natural time-to-get-up-and-time-to-go-to-sleep schedule. This does not bode well for glycemic control, inflammation levels, and overall health stability. Irregular sleep timing—again, even if total sleep hours are adequate—worsens cardiometabolic health, mood, and cognitive resilience.[47, 48, 49] It's just not good.

What's called **chronotype**—your natural propensity for early ("lark") or late ("owl") sleep times—is in part genetic.[50] Misalignment of chronotype with imposed schedules (for example, an evening person forced into 6:00 a.m. starts) results in chronic sleep deficits and circadian stress.[51] Evening chronotypes, in particular, face higher risks of substance abuse and depression as well as obesity and diabetes.[52, 53]

Anchoring a stable wake-up time is going to be your best intervention. The body can adapt bedtimes gradually, but waking at a consistent time—even on weekends—provides a default circadian cue. Morning light further reinforces this rhythm. Misalignment can be adjusted incrementally with bright light exposure and, in some cases, low-dose melatonin at strategic times, but consistency is the master lever to pull you towards the best sleep of your life.

One (More) Thing You Can Do Starting Now: Wake up at the same time every single day, including weekends, no matter what. Even if that means you'll get fewer than 7 to 8 hours of sleep that night . . . sometimes only 6 . . . even only 4. Regardless, that same wake-up time cements your circadian rhythm and prevents "social jetlag"—the discrepancy between social and biological time—so you can get deeper, more restorative sleep long term.[54]

Room Temperature

Did you know that falling asleep is tied to the body's natural cooling process? Core body temperature (CBT) declines in the evening through peripheral vasodilation—heat leaving the core via the skin, especially hands and feet, in other words. This slow but steady temperature decline signals the body to initiate sleep.[55]

So naturally, disruptions in thermoregulation would delay sleep onset and fragment deep sleep. Isn't that interesting. And we want that deep, deep sleep, and unfragmented.

Back to environment. Environmental changes can assist the body's natural cues. A warm shower or bath one to two hours before bed kickstarts that peripheral vasodilation, steepens the CBT decline, and reduces sleep latency.[56] Similarly, warming the extremities with socks or just foot baths helps heat leave the core. According to a meta-analysis by the journal *Neuropsychopharmacology:*

> [H]eat loss, indirectly measured by the distal-proximal skin temperature gradient, was the best predictor variable for sleep onset latency (compared with core body temperature or its rate of change, heart rate, melatonin onset, and subjective sleepiness ratings). The cognitive signal of "lights out" induced relaxation, with a consequent shift in heat redistribution from the core to the periphery (as measured by an abrupt increase in skin temperatures and a rapid fall in heart rate).[57]

An April 2018 study in the *Journal of Physiological Anthropology* disputes the effect on core temperature, but still concludes that warming the feet is beneficial to sleep:

> Feet warming using bed socks during sleep in a cool environment had positive effects on sleep quality by shortened sleep onset, lengthened sleep time, and lessened awakenings during sleep but had no significant influence on core

body temperature . . . [S]leep quality could be improved by manipulation of the foot temperature throughout sleeping.[58]

In the sleep environment itself, an ambient bedroom temperature of 60-67°F (15.5-19°C) correlates with improved sleep depth and efficiency, per the Cleveland Clinic.[59]

For women in menopause, hot flashes and night sweats destabilize CBT, leading to awakenings. Hot flashes are:

> . . . a rapid and exaggerated heat dissipation response, consisting of profuse sweating, peripheral vasodilation, and feelings of intense, internal heat. They are triggered by small elevations in core body temperature (Tc) acting within a greatly reduced thermoneutral zone, i.e., the Tc region between the upper (sweating) and lower (shivering) thresholds. This is due in part, but not entirely, to estrogen depletion at menopause.[60]

Targeted cooling solutions (like thermoregulating mattresses or cooling pads) can help this group, specifically. Per *The Journal of the Menopause Society* in 2022:

> Women who used a cooling mattress pad system experienced significant and clinically meaningful reductions in VMS frequency, sleep disturbance, and hot flash interference

with daily activities over an 8-week period
. . . [A] cooling mattress pad used while
sleeping can provide a nonpharmacological
option to reduce VMS and sleep disturbance
for women experiencing menopausal hot
flashes.[61]

One (More) Thing You Can Do Starting Now:
All I'm asking you to do is to lower your bedroom
temperature to 60 to 68°F (as chilly as you can stand
it) and take a warm bath or shower 1 to 2 hours before
bed every single night, even if it's just 2 to 3 minutes
under the shower head. This will help trigger your body's
natural cooling signal that makes sleep deeper, easier.

Here's how to remember all that. Recently, Dr.
Andrew Huberman had sleep specialist Dr. Matt Walker
on his podcast. Dr. Walker's sleep temperature mantras
were "warm up to cool down to fall asleep" and "stay
cool to stay asleep." As Dr. Walker stated in that very
episode:

[Y]ou have to warm up to cool down to fall
asleep, and I mean warm up in a very specific
way. You have to have the outer surface of
your brain warm up you have to get blood
to the surface of your skin, and that surface
acts like a snake charmer that draws the
warm blood from the core, and it pushes it
to the surface and you radiate the heat out.
And as you radiate the heat out, your core
body temperature plummets.

So why would people be falling asleep in an afternoon meeting when it starts to get a little warm? Well, in part it's because the warmth of the room is drawing the blood out to the surface so what's happening [is that] the core of your brain and your body temperature are starting to drop and at that point that's why you're going to start to feel a little bit more sleepy.[62]

That makes sense to me.

The Not-So-Nervous System

Sleep is orchestrated by the central and autonomic nervous systems. The hypothalamus sets circadian rhythm; the ventrolateral preoptic nucleus (VLPO) inhibits arousal centers through GABA (remember that?). And so the sleep switch gets flipped. The autonomic nervous system shifts from sympathetic dominance (day, alertness) to parasympathetic predominance at night, enabling cardiovascular recovery and immune repair.

Sleep problems can occur when stress keeps the sympathetic system in overdrive. "My mind can't shut off." That's hyperarousal, and not the good kind. According to a February 2010 study in *Sleep Medicine Reviews,* insomnia is a direct consequence of this hyperarousal:

. . . [P]atients with primary insomnia have increased high-frequency EEG activation, abnormal hormone secretion, increased whole body and brain metabolic activation, and elevated heart rate and sympathetic nervous system activation during sleep . . . An animal model that has used odor stress to produce poor sleep in rats has identified specific activated brain sites similar to those found in human brain metabolic studies to suggest that insomnia is a state in which sleep and arousal systems are both simultaneously active.[63]

Sleep may come, but it is light and fragmented. Interventions become necessary in that case to increase the parasympathetic and reduce cortisol output. Like what? Like meditation, controlled breathing, and those warm baths again. Resilience and balance are possible. For meditation, it works by partially mimicking sleep. Per a scientific literature review in *Frontiers in Neurology:*

Many of these [positive, meditation-induced] alterations in physiological functions have great similarities to the changes that are happening during sleep. It has been proposed that sleep is an autoregulatory global phenomenon. It is also true that meditation influences sleep and its functions. It appears that various components of sleep generating mechanisms can be altered with meditation. Meditation, with its global effects on body and brain functions helps to establish a body and mind harmony. Thus meditation practices as an autoregulatory integrated global phenomenon, opens a wider scope for understanding the unique aspects of human sleep and consciousness.[64]

Another practice, controlled breathing, works by activating the parasympathetic nervous system. Per a 2025 scientific literature review in *Frontiers in Sleep:*

> Controlled breathing . . . [fosters] a physiological state conducive to sleep. This autonomic shift leads to reduced heart rate and blood pressure, supporting sleep onset and maintenance. Moreover, breathing exercises help regulate the hypothalamic-pituitary-adrenal (HPA) axis by lowering cortisol levels, reducing stress and anxiety common contributors to insomnia and sleep fragmentation.[65]

And of course, warm baths help your body regulate its temperature which, as discussed by Dr. Walker earlier, affects your ability to sleep. Per the Anchorage Sleep Center:

- Warm baths help promote sleep through a process called **thermoregulation,** which is how the body regulates its internal temperature.

- **Body Temperature Drop** – While a warm bath raises your core body temperature, the real sleep benefit happens when you get out of the tub. As your body cools down, it signals to your brain that it's time for sleep, mimicking the natural drop in body temperature that occurs at night.

- **Melatonin Production** – The cooling effect after a bath helps trigger the release of melatonin, the hormone that regulates sleep.

- **Muscle Relaxation** – Warm water helps relax tight muscles and relieve tension, making it easier for your body to unwind before bed.

- **Stress Reduction** – Soaking in warm water has been shown to reduce cortisol, the stress hormone, and activate the parasympathetic nervous system, which promotes relaxation.[66]

One (More) Thing You Can Do Starting Now: Adopt a nightly parasympathetic activation ritual—deep breathing (I suggest the 4-7-8 method of 4-second inhale, 7-second hold, 8-second exhale), mindfulness, or a warm bath—to calm the nervous system and turn off stress before bed. Stress is not (just) an issue of the mind; it's of the nervous system. Change your physical state and mental state, change your sleep.

Let There Be Light (Then None at All)

If wake-up time is the little hand of your circadian clockface, light is the big hand. Retinal light signals (meaning light entering through your retinas) reach the suprachiasmatic nucleus (SCN), which synchronizes the body's internal clock. *It is light; therefore, time to be awake and alert.* Morning light suppresses melatonin and triggers cortisol release. Per the *Journal of Clinical Endocrinology and Metabolism* in 2001, "The early morning transition from dim to bright light suppressed melatonin secretion, induced an immediate, greater than 50% elevation of cortisol levels, and limited the deterioration of alertness normally associated with overnight sleep deprivation."[67]

A 2023 study in the journal *Life* found similar:

> . . . [E]xposure to bright lights of any colour during the late night or early morning can induce significant increases in cortisol secretion relative to time-matched dim light comparison conditions. Furthermore, exposure to bright lights with stronger short-wavelength (blue/green) components in the early morning typically induced greater increases in cortisol relative to lights with stronger long-wavelength (red) components. Thus, the circadian regulation of cortisol is sensitive to the wavelength composition of environmental lighting, in line with the more commonly studied melatonin.[68]

Evening light, however—even at everyday indoor levels with a few lights and screens on at home—delays melatonin and promotes wakefulness.[69] Even dim light during sleep can raise heart rate, blunt insulin sensitivity, and shallow out otherwise deep sleep, per a 2022 PNAS study.[70]

All this physiological cascade, simply due to unnecessary additional light. You're basically telling your body and brain, *It is (still) light; therefore, (still) time to be awake and alert.*

As you might imagine, not-enough daytime light slows your circadian rhythms. You'll feel tired in the morning and into the afternoon, then buzzed at night by the time your body has finally woken up.

My prescription is simple. Get bright light exposure in the morning (preferably outdoors) and minimize artificial lights at night. Darkness signals melatonin to rise so sleepiness overtakes you. If unavoidable, very low-intensity red light is the least disruptive. Get blue light blockers as well.

One (More) Thing You Can Do Starting Now: Get outside for bright morning sunlight, and keep your sleep environment as dark as possible at night. A sleep mask is suggested; blackout curtains are preferred.

The Metabolism Connection

I introduced this relationship above. Sleep and metabolism are two strands of a tight cord that cannot be untangled. As stated by the *Journal of Clinical Endocrinology in 2010,* "Poor sleep worsens insulin resistance and appetite regulation; meanwhile, late-in-the-day and ultraprocessed meals fragment sleep."[71] Furthermore, fat-heavy and unduly spicy dinners elevate core body temperature and disturb digestion. Regarding high-fat dinners, a 2016 study in the journal *Nutrition* found:

> Fluctuation of sleep duration over 5 y was observed with an increase in short-duration sleepers (<7 h) and a decrease in long-duration sleepers (9 h). The highest quartile of fat intake from dinner at baseline was associated with persistent short sleep over 5 y . . . The highest quartile of fat intake from breakfast at baseline was associated with less falling asleep during the day at follow up (odds ratio 0.36, 95% confidence interval 0.14–0.94, P for trend 0.006). Dinner fat intake at baseline was not associated with short sleep (<7 h) at follow up.[72]

For spicy dinners, Johns Hopkins Medicine has this warning for us:

> Eating spicy foods can cause heartburn, which can impact your sleep, says Johns Hopkins sleep expert Charlene E. Gamaldo, M.D. And when you lie down, that acid reflux often worsens. If you have sleep apnea, your symptoms may worsen, too, if the backed-up acid irritates your airway.
>
> What's more, research shows that consuming red pepper can increase your core body temperature, which is disruptive since core body temperature naturally drops during sleep. (Being overheated can make it more

difficult for the body to make this temperature transition.)

For better sleep: Avoid spicy foods within three hours of bedtime. Do the same with tomato sauce and other acidic foods if they give you heartburn or indigestion.[73]

We mustn't interpret this data to imply a light last meal of the day is a better alternative. Going to bed hungry (or with low blood sugar) can also trigger cortisol surges that wake you up. Carolinas Thyroid Institute explains the problem:

> People with hypoglycemia tend to have difficulty making the right amount of cortisol at the right times of the day or night. They also have blood sugar levels that spike and then crash throughout the day. If they go too long without eating they experience lightheadedness, irritability, shakiness, a spacey feeling, and other symptoms that signify the brain is not getting enough glucose.
>
> In these cases, not only does blood sugar drop too low during the night, but the adrenal glands don't produce enough cortisol to keep the brain fueled. In response, the body sounds the emergency alarm by releasing "fight-or-flight" hormones. These stress hormones raise blood sugar back to a safer level. Unfortunately, they also raise stress, which

can cause anxiety or panic in the middle of the night. Hence the waking up at 3 a.m. and not being able to fall back asleep.[74]

As you can see, the cord is tight. What we can take away from all this—among other tentative conclusions—is that meal timing is critical. Finish dinner at least 2 to 3 hours before bed. A moderate, balanced meal with protein, complex carbs, and healthy fats stabilizes glucose.[75] Contrary to some fads, carbohydrates at dinner can aid sleep by helping tryptophan cross into the brain.[76] That said, although carbohydrates can help tryptophan make this passage, this process only occurs with such low levels of protein that it's not relevant to a normal diet.[77] Still, you must avoid late-night snacking. (I'll talk more about the nutrition essentials of middle age in Chapter 4.)

Again, and no surprise, but stimulants and alcohol fall into the no-no category as well. Caffeine blocks adenosine and disrupts deep sleep even six hours after intake.[78, 79] Alcohol induces drowsiness but fragments REM and increases nighttime awakenings.[80, 81] Avoid both before bed.

One (More) Thing You Can Do Starting Now: Eat your last substantial meal 2 to 3 hours before bedtime so your blood sugar has time to stabilize. Set yourself up for deeper, more restorative sleep.

Breathe Better, Sleep Better

Good sleep depends on uninterrupted breathing and

proper oxygen levels. Obstructive sleep apnea (OSA) is common yet often undiagnosed in your fifties and beyond. OSA prevalence is four times higher in older adults than in younger adults less than 40.[82] A study in the *American Journal of Respiratory and Critical Care Medicine* found that OSA occurs in 4.7 percent of adults between the ages of 45 and 64 (versus 1.2 percent for those younger than 45.)[83] A 2025 study in the journal *Sleep Medicine* states that an estimated 80 percent of people with OSA remain undiagnosed.[84] Repeated pauses in breathing drops oxygen causes wake-ups so you can, somewhat consciously, breathe more air into your lungs.

But even without full apnea, nasal congestion or chronic mouth breathing can fragment sleep through the night, keep you out of that all-precious REM, and worsen fatigue day in and day out. According to a 2005 study in the *European Respiratory Journal:*

> Patients . . . experienced significant improvements in sleep architecture (improved sleep efficiency, less stage 1 sleep and more stage 2 sleep, slow-wave sleep and REM sleep) during the active treatment night . . . despite a relatively modest improvement in sleep apnoea severity with the active treatment. Others have also demonstrated a reduction in sleep fragmentation with treatment of nasal obstruction, even in the absence of any significant improvement in sleep apnoea severity.[85]

Regarding fatigue, the *Journal of Allergy and Clinical Immunology* states in a study that:

> . . . [S]elf-reported chronic symptoms of rhinitis were significantly related to excessive daytime sleepiness and not feeling rested regardless of amount of sleep. Sleep-disordered breathing, including habitual snoring, is related to hypersomnolence; therefore, associations between rhinitis and sleepiness may be explained by sleep-disordered breathing. However, it is possible that rhinitis symptoms, independent of their effect on breathing, may cause cortical arousal and fragmented sleep . . . [S]omnolence due to sleep fragmentation may be compounded by sleepiness caused by daytime use of medication.[86]

Sleep screening thus becomes essential. We do a 30-day sleep study in most of our patients at Velocity, and we've found a lot of previously undiagnosed OSA. Loud snoring, gasping, or heavily-fatigued waking are warning signs. Treatments range from CPAP and oral devices to simple steps like side sleeping, nasal rinses, and breathing strips. Even small changes—like clearing nasal passages before bed—can improve oxygenation. This is what you want.

One (More) Thing You Can Do Starting Now: If you snore or feel exhausted despite "enough" sleep, get screened for sleep apnea. Airway freedom is life-changing.

The Gut-Brain-Sleep Axis

The gut-brain axis is real, and it really matters for good-quality sleep. Most serotonin (the precursor to melatonin) is produced in the gastrointestinal tract, and dysbiosis or inflammation can divert tryptophan away from sleep hormones. Leaky gut and cytokines like IL-6 or TNF-α also sabotage rest. Poor gut health, unsurprisingly, correlates with insomnia, anxiety, and depression.[87] Conversely, high-fiber diets and probiotics can improve sleep quality and reduce night wakings (in addition, fiber supports certain dietary strategies, such as the cardiac health and longevity protocol you'll be reading about in Chapter 4). Addressing reflux, IBS, or intolerances can also remove hidden sleep disruptors. According to a 2024 paper in the journal *Nutrients*:

> Butyrate, one of the [short chain fatty acids] produced by the microbiota, is also naturally present in dairy products such as milk, butter, and cheese. Butyrate is readily absorbed into the portal circulation and transported to the liver. This is evidenced by the concentration gradient between systemic and portal butyrate concentrations. Administration of tributyrin, an ester composed of three molecules of butyric acid and glycerol, to mice resulted in a nearly 50% increase in non-rapid eye movement (NREM) sleep for four hours, confirming that butyrate may act as a signaling molecule that induces sleep.[88]

In other words, the gut microbiota directly affect sleep in mice. But the study doesn't merely stop at the rodents:

> . . . [H]igher SCFA levels in feces are observed in obese individuals and those with sleep problems, which may be caused by gut microbiota dysbiosis and impaired intestinal barrier permeability. Consequently, it is proposed that maintaining a healthy gut microbiota has a considerable impact on sleep quality.
>
> . . . Research indicates that changes in the composition of the gut microbiota are observed in individuals with sleep disorders. In patients with insomnia, a reduction in the abundance of bacteria responsible for the metabolism of dietary fiber to SCFAs can be observed, while SCFAs may have a beneficial effect on sleep duration.[89]

All of that is to say that your gut has a direct effect on your brain, and thus your sleep quality, which makes sense because it's all part of the same body.

One (More) Thing You Can Do Starting Now: Support gut health with a diverse, fiber-rich diet and probiotics. Your microbiome directly influences your sleep hormones and recovery. As goes belly, so goes brain!

No Technoference

Modern bedrooms are cluttered with invisible and visible disruptors, like EMFs, Wi-Fi, electronics, hums, vibrations, and blue light. Electromagnetic exposure can suppress melatonin, though per a 2013 study in *Radiation Protection Dosimetry,* this claim is somewhat disputed.[90] But we do know for sure that it increases nighttime brain arousal. According to a study in *NeuroReport:*

> Healthy, young male subjects were exposed for 30 min to EMF (900 MHz; spatial peak specific absorption rate 1 W/kg) during the waking period preceding sleep. Compared with the control condition with sham exposure, spectral power of the EEG in non-rapid eye movement sleep was increased . . . [E]xposure during waking modifies the EEG during subsequent sleep. Thus the changes of brain function induced by pulsed high-frequency EMF outlast the exposure period.[91]

Now, whether or not EMFs are indeed the culprit, this stands: Interference in the sleep environment—gadgets, screens, notifications—keeps the body on alert. Reducing "technoference" reduces the temptation to scroll or work late regardless. The Sleep Foundation explains why:

> The biological clock in healthy adults follows a 24-hour sleep-wake cycle. When the sun rises in the morning, your body produces

cortisol, a hormone that makes you feel awake and alert. As daylight fades, the body releases another hormone, melatonin, that produces feelings of sleepiness.

Electronic back-lit devices like cell phones, tablets, readers, and computers emit short-wavelength enriched light, also known as blue light. Fluorescent and LED lights also emit blue light, which has been shown to reduce or delay the natural production of melatonin in the evening and decrease feelings of sleepiness. Blue light can also reduce the amount of time you spend in slow-wave and rapid-eye movement (REM) sleep, two stages of the sleep cycle that are vital for cognitive functioning.[92]

One (More) Thing You Can Do Starting Now: Make your bedroom a tech-free sanctuary. Remove electronics, keep Wi-Fi off at night, and reserve the bed for sleep and physical intimacy only.

Ritual, Routine, and Rest

Bedtime rituals create powerful conditioned responses. As with children and a bedtime story before sleep, adults benefit from consistent cues, like smells, sounds, and sequences of behaviors that signal it's time to shut down for the night. According to a 2020 study in *Applied Physiology, Nutrition, and Metabolism*, while exact thresholds are hard to determine, ". . . the available evidence supports that earlier sleep timing and regularity in sleep patterns with consistent bedtimes and wake-up times are favourably associated with health."[93]

As additional solutions, lavender aromatherapy, calm sounds like ASMR or ambient nature-themed music, and repeated pre-sleep prep steps (dim lights, pajamas, journaling, quiet reading) train the brain to expect rest.[94, 95, 96, 97] Over time, these cues alone can induce drowsiness. On the other hand, negative triggers—like checking email in bed—train the opposite association. *Oh, the bed? That's my second office.* Not good!

One (More) Thing You Can Do Starting Now: Build a simple bedtime ritual using multisensory cues, i.e., smell, sound, and touch. Repeat nightly to train your body and brain for sleep basically on command.

All Together Now . . .

To review, your ten takeaways to conduct your perfect Sleep Symphony are as follows:

1. **Hormones**: Dim lights and cut screens 2 hours before bed so melatonin rises and cortisol falls.
2. **Sleep Timing**: Wake up at the same time every day, weekends included.
3. **Temperature**: Keep your bedroom 60-68°F and take a warm bath/shower 1 to 2 hours before bed.
4. **Nervous System**: Do a nightly parasympathetic ritual (breathing, mindfulness, or warm bath).
5. **Light Environment**: Get morning sunlight, and make your bedroom pitch-dark at night.
6. **Metabolism**: Finish dinner 2 to 3 hours before

bed; no late snacking, caffeine, or booze.

7. **Oxygenation**: If you snore or wake tired, get screened for sleep apnea and clear your airway.

8. **Gut Health**: Eat a fiber-rich diet or probiotics; a healthy microbiome means deeper sleep.

9. **Interference**: Make your bedroom tech-free: no Wi-Fi, no electronics, just sleep (and intimacy).

10. **Routine**: Build a nightly ritual (lavender, calming sounds, journaling, dim lights).

How did implementing this sort of intervention set work out for our heroine Laura? Let's see.

Laura's Story, Continued

Laura's better-sleep progress wasn't instant once she started making changes. For the first few weeks, she struggled to break old patterns. She'd slip back into scrolling or pour herself that late-night drink. Just a half glass. OK, just another half. OK, one more sip. From the bottle. *Gulp.*

But we kept bringing Laura back to her "why"— her kids, her father, her own health. And slowly, the routine changed. Two months into the new protocol, she was sleeping through the night for the first time in years. Three months in, she woke up with more energy than she thought possible. And that energy unlocked everything else. She started cooking healthier meals with her teenagers. She signed up for a yoga class and actually had the energy to go. Her joint pain eased as the weight began to come off—a remarkable 10 whole percent of her body weight disappeared in six months.

Her A1C dropped from pre-diabetic levels to below 5 percent, officially taking her out of diabetic risk territory.

These numbers, as impressive as they are, tell only part of the story. For Laura, the real transformation was emotional, relational, even spiritual. For the first time in years, she felt present. As in, present with her kids, cooking meals and exercising together. Present with her father, bringing both care and companionship. Present at work, no longer dragging herself through meetings on watery coffee fumes. And of course . . . present with herself. No more self-numbing with wine and screens. Finally resting. Reflecting. Recharging.

She often says now, "I didn't realize how different I could feel once I was actually fully rested."

That single shift—choosing sleep as the foundation of Laura's health—kickstarted a virtuous cycle. Better rest led to better food choices. More energy led to regular movement. Lower stress made her more patient with her teenagers and more emotionally available to her father. More than anything, Laura felt like herself again. And for the first time in a long time. For the first time since her dad got sick. For the first time since . . . kids. Laura, like Robert, felt like a new person. For some such a change takes newfound purpose, for others it's putting sleep first.

The best days really do start the night before.

CHAPTER 4
Upgrade Your Nutrition

Samantha and Daniel live separate lives. They never met. They don't even share the same life stage. But their stories echo across one another in ways that matter for you. Two lives, two phases, one theme—nutrition as both mirror and lever.

Samantha was a wellness blogger, the kind with thousands of readers eager to know what was in her smoothie this week. She had "tried it all"—keto, intermittent fasting, gut cleanses, carb-heavy resets. Her audience loved the experimentation. But privately, she felt no better.

She was simply yo-yo-ing. She would go back and forth, trying all sorts of different things, people pulling her one direction or another. When we got her at Velocity, she was on the fasting kick. Now in Daniel's case, that made all the sense in the world. But for Samantha, we don't recommend fasting when women are enduring the hormonal changes of menopause. In fact, it probably wrecked her even more, which is the part her followers didn't see. From the mid-afternoon crashes and brain fog to the irritability that crept into family life and the weight that wouldn't stay off. The bloating that made her clothes fit differently week to week.

She came to Velocity Health not as an influencer but as a woman finally admitting she needed a more comprehensive approach. As she put it, she was "kind of all over the place." Samantha had been taking upwards of fifty different vitamins and supplements by the time she came to us, which is not uncommon. Sometimes, dieters are on a huge cocktail of supplements and powders. They want and need guidance.

Guidance means data—like labs, a DEXA scan, a continuous glucose monitor. Samantha's results shocked her. The picture-perfect smoothie she'd been posting spiked her blood sugar sky-high. Some of her supplements were taxing her liver, inflaming it, nudging her toward prediabetes even though technically she wasn't there yet. Her visceral fat—the hidden kind that wraps around organs—was higher than expected. She was what the literature calls "normal weight obese," or skinny-fat. Her insulin resistance score was creeping up also. All the hidden cost of years chasing every diet trend at once. Samantha wasn't failing; the advice was failing her.

Daniel, on the other hand, was a new dad in his early forties, with thirty extra pounds around his middle and a doctor's note warning him about prediabetes. He was busy with career, occupied with family, and honest about being lost. He reminded me of my friends at this phase of life. We're all in our forties, and we all have kids 5 to 6 and under. We look back and realize we've gained forty pounds, *used to be* athletic, and now feel self-conscious that we can't move how we used to.

Daniel's turning point was fatherhood. Like Robert, his mind was on his legacy. His kids and grandkids. He needed to be as good as he possibly could for as long as he could.

Daniel had consumed the same flood of health advice as Samantha. He'd seen Peter Attia, Andrew Huberman, the endless podcasts, the ☐ threads. He was even considering cold plunges and saunas. But where could he go with all this stuff? What would work and what wouldn't?

What Daniel needed was a clear plan. Intermittent fasting worked for him because of his biology, not because it was trendy. A high-protein diet, paired with resistance training, began to reshape his body. He cut alcohol, stopped smoking weed, and recommitted to the gym. He even opted to self-administer research peptides—a sophisticated cocktail of GLP-1 and growth hormone analogs—that accelerated fat loss and muscle gain.

While I'm not recommending that level of experimentation for everyone, I will recommend you take seriously similar nutrition strategies as those I advised Daniel and Samantha to follow. Here's what all that looks like for you.

The Fork in the Road

Every diet has a study. Paleo has them. Vegan has them. Carnivore has them. Keto has them. Mediterranean has them. If you look hard enough, you'll find a "proof" that your favorite approach is the answer. That's part of the problem.

Every single person reading this has been exposed to dietary advice—on TV, in the doctor's office, from a podcast, in the aisle at Whole Foods—and whether you realize it or not, you've internalized it. It's baked into how you shop, how you cook, and what you believe food can or cannot do for you. But how much of that advice is real?

For decades, mainstream nutrition advice has been not advice but advertising. Food companies lobby for labels like "heart healthy," "low fat," "whole grain," and "low cholesterol," which sound authoritative but are often nothing more than marketing claims. Remember the "low-fat" craze of the 1980s and 1990s? It was supposed to solve heart disease and obesity. Instead, it ushered in an era of ultra-processed, high-carb products that left people sicker and heavier than ever. According to a 2022 study in the journal *Nutrients*, "[t]here is strong evidence that consumption of SSBs leads to higher energy intake and more weight gain. A similar pattern is also seen with other UPFs."[98] With regards to obesity trends, the the study found as follows:

> The prevalence of obesity in American adults (age 20–74, both genders) rose from 15.0% in 1976–1980, to 23.3% in 1988–1994, and to 30.9% in 1999–2000. What is especially noteworthy is that this fast-rising prevalence among American adults was similar in all age groups, in both men and women, and in

all major ethnic groups including Caucasian Americans, African Americans, and Mexican Americans. This rise in the prevalence of obesity continued in both genders during the period 1999 to 2016.[99]

Consider next the so-called war on cholesterol: Egg yolks and red meat were vilified for decades based on shaky science. Per a 2015 study in the journal *Nutrients*:

> The 1968 American Heart Association announced a dietary recommendation that all individuals consume less than 300 mg of dietary cholesterol per day and no more than three whole eggs per week. This recommendation has not only significantly impacted the dietary patterns of the population, but also resulted in the public limiting a highly nutritious and affordable source of high quality nutrients, including choline which was limited in the diets of most individuals. The egg industry addressed the egg issue with research documenting the minimal effect of egg intake on plasma lipoprotein levels, as well as research verifying the importance of egg nutrients in a variety of issues related to health promotion. In 2015 dietary cholesterol and egg restrictions have been dropped by most health promotion agencies worldwide and recommended to be dropped from the 2015 Dietary Guidelines for Americans.[100]

Regarding red meat being unhealthy, we have correlation mistaken for causation. A 2020 study in *Critical Reviews in Food Science and Nutrition* states that:

> It has been shown that Western-style meat eating is closely associated with nutrient-poor diets, obesity, smoking, and limited physical activity. Given the fact that health authorities have been intensely promoting the view that meat is unhealthy, health-conscious people may be inclined to reduce intake.[101]

Meanwhile, the real culprits—refined carbs and sugar—were largely ignored. A 2004 study in the *American Journal of Clinical Nutrition*, focusing on the period between 1980 and 1997, associates sugar, and especially corn syrup (a common additive to many snack foods), with Type 2 diabetes.[102] It may thus (or may not) come as a surprise that sugar has a greater role to play than fat in cardiovascular risk. According to a 2010 study in the *American Journal of Clinical Nutrition*:

> For several decades, the diet-heart paradigm that high intake of saturated fat and cholesterol increases the risk of atherosclerosis and ischemic heart disease (IHD) has been the driving force behind national and international dietary recommendations for prevention of IHD. This model, which promotes diets that are typically low in fat (particularly saturated fat) and high in complex carbohydrates, has

led to substantial decline in the percentage of energy intake from total and saturated fats in the United States. At the same time, it has spurred a compensatory increase in consumption of refined carbohydrates and added sugars—a dietary shift that may be contributing to the current twin epidemics of obesity and diabetes.

. . . A recent pooled analysis of 11 American and European cohort studies (n = 344,696 persons) found no association between decreased risk of IHD and replacement of saturated fat with carbohydrates; indeed, the approach was associated with a slightly increased risk. Similarly, a meta-analysis of 21 cohort studies (n = 347,747 subjects) found no significant association between intake of saturated fat compared with carbohydrates and risk of IHD, stroke, and total cardiovascular events . Conversely, observational studies as well as randomized clinical trials show that substitution of polyunsaturated for saturated fat has a beneficial effect on IHD.[103]

The confusion is structural. Nutrition is notoriously difficult to study. You can't lock someone in some kind of metabolic ward for twenty-five years and control every bite they eat. At best, researchers rely on self-reported food diaries (e.g., "What did you eat last month?"), which are unreliable.[104] How many of you can remember what you ate yesterday? Or last week? Anyway, most long-term studies are likewise observational; they can suggest correlations but can't prove cause and effect. The randomized controlled trials that do exist are usually small, short, and contradictory. As a 2022 study in the *International Journal of Epidemiology* states:

> Nutritional epidemiology is criticized for its inability to provide plausible information on the causal effects of diet on health and disease outcomes, a key to both scientific understanding and guiding public policies. Although most public dietary guidelines globally have arrived at similar conclusions, they all continue to rely strongly on observational studies. It is well known in epidemiology that observational study settings produce the lowest-quality data with perceivable but also unidentifiable confounding and with very limited, if any, opportunities to assess direct causality. However, we would hope for the same reliability for nutritional recommendations as for pharmacological treatments—only substances known to have causal effects should be recommended and used . . . Low compliance and high dropout rates are also common in nutrition studies if participants are asked to change their typical diets for more than a few months . . . There is also rarely a placebo group with zero intake of a certain nutrient.[105]

And this is why every "diet tribe" can point to a paper that backs them up. The vegans have their data. The carnivores have theirs. Keto has meta-analyses. Mediterranean is practically canonized by the American Heart Association. But none of these prove one-size-fits-all truth. They prove only that *something* works for *someone* and *some* of the time. The Mediterranean diet is said to fight against chronic health problems, but in 2018 a landmark study that allegedly proved the diet's benefits was retracted.[106, 107] Keto helps control diabetes, but may also increase cholesterol beyond ideal levels, thus potentially posing cardiovascular risks.[108, 109] The Paleo diet is said to help with weight loss, but the benefits of the diet are also stated to be a side effect of cutting out processed foods, making it hard to conclude whether the Paleo diet actually helped.[110, 111] Vegan diets are claimed to fight cardiovascular problems (as a lot of diets do), but it can also increase the risk of bone fractures.[112, 113]

Here's my conclusion on the matter: **There is no single diet that works for everyone.** Genetics, age, sex, hormones, activity levels, stress, sleep, and even gut microbiome diversity all change how your body processes food. For some, intermittent fasting unlocks weight loss and clarity. For others—particularly perimenopausal women—it can worsen fatigue, cravings, and hormonal imbalance. The same diet can be a miracle for one person and a disaster for another.

Still, there are universal principles. A real, whole-food diet beats a processed one every time. Ultra-processed food—what most of us eat far too much of—wreaks havoc on insulin sensitivity, metabolic health, and long-term risk of chronic disease. And most people, regardless of their "diet tribe," overeat refined carbohydrates while undereating protein. That's why, in our clinic, we measure insulin resistance markers all day, every day. Because unless you're actively managing insulin, you're flying blind.

So the real question isn't, *What's the best diet?* It's, *What's your goal?* Do you want to lose fat while preserving muscle? Do you want to gain lean mass and strength? Are you focused on stabilizing energy for long workdays and sharp decision-making? Are you trying to prevent diabetes, dementia, or cardiovascular disease because they run in your family? Each of these points toward a different set of nutritional priorities.

Nutrition is your fuel. And just like fuel in a car, the type and amount you need depends on what kind of engine you have and how hard you're running it. A professional athlete, a new mom, and a sixty-year-old executive all require different strategies to get the best performance out of their bodies.

Once you match your nutrition to your biology and your goals, everything gets easier. Energy stabilizes. Labs improve. Fat loss or muscle gain stops being a mystery. You stop yo-yoing between trends and finally feel confident that the food you're eating is the right fuel for you. That's where we're going next—to the Velocity Nutrition Strategy.

The Velocity Nutrition Strategy

Like I said, let's start with your specific goals, then work our way down to specific meals, both at home and out and about. Begin.

1. Choose the primary objective (one only at start).

- **Fat loss** (you don't just "lose weight"; fat loss is the result of eating in a daily calorie deficit, consuming satiating meals, and keeping cortisol in check)

- **Metabolic rehabilitation** (reversing prediabetes and/or insulin resistance)

- **Body recomposition** (this means noticeable muscle gain and is the result of higher protein intake and progressive overload workouts)

- **Cognitive wellness and energy stability** (brain fog and low mojo are addressed by balanced blood sugar and anti-inflammatory foods)

- **Gut repair** (the best way to heal the gastrointestinal tract is giving it a break, i.e., food elimination and slow reintroductions)

- **Cardiac health and longevity** (priority foods will be those that lower ApoB, blood pressure, and weight)

2. Apply constraints (e.g., dietary restrictions, medical conditions, etc.).

- **Medical conditions:** chronic kidney disease, thyroid issues, gallbladder dysfunction, gout, certain medications.

- **Life stage:** perimenopause, menopause, andropause.

- **Ethical preferences:** vegan, vegetarian.

- **Allergy:** gluten-free, dairy-free.

- **Logistics:** travel schedule, cooking time, budget, family members.

- **Performance:** training for endurance activities, regular weightlifting, other strenuous physical exercise or hobbies.

3. Run your numbers (see below).

Once you set your intention and you layer on any additional factors that would affect your recommended dietary plan going forwards, you're ready to calculate *how much* you should eat. From there, we'll get to the *what*. But first, we'll deal with *how much*. On to macros and timing.

Based on your chosen goal in bullet 1, use your ideal body weight to calculate your necessary macro profile.

<u>Note</u>: Below, you are going to see the word "maintenance."

This is the number of calories to eat daily so you stay your same weight, neither losing nor gaining. The best way to really know this daily number for you is by getting a resting metabolic rate (RMR) done using a calorimeter and then adding any NEAT and EAT to that. What are NEAT and EAT? I'm glad you asked. **NEAT** stands for **N**on-**E**xercise **A**ctivity **T**hermogenesis. This is all the energy you burn from daily movement that isn't "formal" exercise. Think walking around the office, fidgeting, standing, doing chores, even pacing while on the phone. NEAT can vary hugely from person to person and is often the hidden factor in why one person maintains their weight on 2,800 calories while another does so on 2,000. An example of this variability can be seen with observing obese people. A low level of NEAT is associated with obesity.[114] According to the American Heart Association, obese individuals compound their condition by becoming even more sedentary than leaner people:

> Evidence suggests that low NEAT may occur in obesity but in a very specific fashion. Obese individuals appear to exhibit an innate tendency to be seated for 2.5 hours per day more than sedentary lean counterparts. If obese individuals were to adopt the lean "NEAT-o-type," they could potentially expend an additional 350 kcal per day.[115]

As you might expect, in contrast to NEAT, **EAT** stands for **E**xercise **A**ctivity **T**hermogenesis. This is the energy you burn from intentional workouts, like lifting weights, running, cycling, swimming, classes, sports, you name it. EAT is the most obvious calorie burn to track, but it's actually NEAT that usually makes the bigger difference over time. An active lifestyle is just that . . . a *lifestyle*. Not a little time in the gym, on the treadmill, or with the weights a little each day surrounded by a sedentary lifestyle at all other hours. According to PLOS One in a 2013 study, an hour of daily exercise is not enough to offset an otherwise sedentary way of life.[116]

This means that when it comes to physical activity, you have to move around more in general, not just when you're at the gym.

All together, RMR, NEAT, and EAT give you your true **maintenance calories**. That's the daily target where your body does *not* gain *or* lose fat *or* muscle. Once you know it, you can adjust upward (to build) or downward (to lose) with precision.

For the purposes of simplicity in the section below—and for speed, frankly—we are going to use your ideal body weight in pounds multiplied by 10 and 12 to give you a two-number starting range if your priority is either fat loss or metabolic rehabilitation. These beat NEAT in terms of intuitiveness but give you roughly the same information. Let's run those numbers in the context of your specific goal below.

Fat loss OR metabolic rehabilitation

- **Calories:** *Ideal* BW(lb) × 10-12
- **Protein:** 0.9-1.0 g/lb (2.0-2.2 g/kg)
- **Carbs:** 50-125 g/day to start (lower end if CGM >160 mg/dL often)
- **Fat:** remainder
- **Timing: 30-50 g protein at breakfast; carbs earlier in day/around training; stop eating ≥3 h before bed.**

Body rerecomposition

- **Calories:** Maintenance + 5-10% extra
- **Protein:** 0.8-1.4 g/lb
- **Carbs:** 1.0-1.4 g/lb (taper on off days)
- **Fat:** 20-30% kcals
- **Timing:** Majority of carbs peri-workout; last meal low-fat/moderate protein for sleep quality.

Cognitive wellness and energy stability

- **Calories:** Maintenance
- **Protein:** 0.8-1.0 g/lb
- **Carbs:** 100-175 g/day from low-GI plants/ berries/legumes
- **Fat:** Emphasize EVOO, avocado, nuts, omega-3s
- **Timing:** 12:12 eating window; largest meal midday

Gut repair

- **Calories:** Maintenance or slightly below (consider intermittent fasting, but avoid aggressive deficits during healing)
- **Protein:** 0.7.-1g/lb
- **Carbs:** 75-125g/day, focus on low-FODMAP vegetables, squash, cooked root vegetables, white rice; avoid fermentable triggers initially
- **Fat:** Remainder, but favor soothing anti-inflammatory fats (EVOO, avocado, omega-3s, MCT if tolerated)
- **Timing:**
- Begin with food elimination (gluten, dairy, high-FODMAP, processed oils)
- Reintroduce foods one at a time every 3-5 days

- Meal frequency: 2-3 calm, non-hurried meals; avoid grazing

- Extras: Bone broth, L-glutamine (5 g BID), zinc carnosine, probiotics (start with single-strain or spore-based), digestive bitters/enzymes

Cardiac health and longevity:

- **Calories:** Maintenance (avoid large surpluses, consider occasional fasting)

- **Protein:** 0.8-1.0 g/lb, with high emphasis on tyrosine-rich foods (fish, poultry, eggs) and tryptophan sources for serotonin balance

- **Carbs:** 100-175 g/day, primarily low-GI vegetables, berries, legumes, sweet potatoes, quinoa; avoid refined sugar spikes

- **Fat:** 35-45% kcals, prioritize DHA/EPA (fatty fish or algal oil), EVOO, nuts, avocado, phospholipid-rich foods (egg yolk, krill oil)

- **Timing:**

- 12:12 eating window or early TRF (e.g., 8a-6p)

- Largest meal midday for stable focus

- Avoid heavy meals within 3 hours of bed

4. Make your shopping list.

The following foods (and food categories) are some examples of those I recommend in order to get you a complete nutritional profile consistent with only a diet of real, whole foods.

- **Proteins:** eggs/egg whites, chicken breast/thigh, turkey, lean beef/bison, salmon/sardines, tuna pouches, shrimp, Greek/Skyr yogurt, cottage cheese, tofu/tempeh, edamame, protein powder (whey or plant), deli turkey (no sugar), canned beans/lentils.

- **Veg (non-starchy):** spinach/spring mix, arugula, broccoli, cauliflower, asparagus, green beans, cucumbers, peppers, mushrooms, onions, sauerkraut/kimchi.

- **Carbs (starchy/fruit):** potatoes/sweet potatoes, rice (incl. parboiled), quinoa, oats/steel-cut, berries, apples, bananas, legumes, corn/tortillas (GF if needed).

- **Fats:** extra-virgin olive oil, avocado/guac, olives, nuts (pistachio/almond/walnut), nut butter, chia/flax, ghee.

- **Flavor & pantry:** salsa, mustard, hot sauce, tamari/coconut aminos, lemon, herbs/spices, broth, low-sugar marinara, pickles.

- **Convenience:** microwave rice cups, frozen veg steamers, pre-washed greens, rotisserie chicken (plain), frozen salmon burgers, single-serve guac/hummus.

5. Know your menus.

Here are sample suggested menus for breakfast, lunch,

and dinner with three options each for a total of nine meals. Review the list below for your primary objective you selected in step 1. Then adjust as needed based on additional dietary considerations, if any, from step 2.

Goal: Fat loss

Breakfast (30-45 g protein)

1. Omelet: 3 eggs + 3 egg whites, spinach, mushrooms, feta (dairy-free: skip feta), ½ avocado. (gluten-free/low-carb OK; vegan: tofu scramble)
2. Greek bowl: 1 cup 0% Greek yogurt (DF: coconut yogurt + plant protein), 1 scoop protein powder, ½ cup berries, 1 tbsp chia.
3. Savory plate: smoked salmon 4-5 oz, tomatoes, cucumbers, olives, drizzle EVOO; 1 slice GF high-protein bread or none.

Lunch (35-45 g protein)

1. High-protein salad: 6-8 oz grilled chicken, big greens, non-starchy veg, EVOO + lemon; optional ½ cup chickpeas (skip if CGM >160).
2. Turkey roll-ups: 6-8 oz deli turkey, pickles, mustard, side: raw veg + guac; add fruit only if CGM stable.
3. Tofu stir-fry: 8 oz tofu, broccoli/peppers, coconut aminos; optional ½ cup cauliflower rice.

Dinner (35-50 g protein)

1. Salmon (6-8 oz), roasted asparagus + cauliflower, ½ small potato if CGM allows (else double veg).
2. Lean beef/bison (6 oz) lettuce-wrap tacos, pico, avocado; side slaw.
3. Shrimp zucchini "noodles" with garlic, olive oil, herbs; parmesan optional (DF skip).

Restrictions swaps:

- **GF:** Use potatoes/rice/lettuce wraps; tamari/coconut aminos vs soy.

- **DF:** Coconut yogurt; EVOO/ghee; no cheese.

- **Veg:** Tofu/tempeh/edamame; add plant protein powder; watch legume portions for CGM.

- **Low-carb:** Replace starch with extra veg; add 1-2 tbsp olive oil or ½ avocado.

Goal: Metabolic rehabilitation

Breakfast

1. Protein oats: ½ cup oats cooked + 1 scoop whey, ½ banana, 1 tbsp peanut butter. (GF: GF oats; DF: plant protein)
2. Eggs & fruit: 3 eggs, side berries + ½ cup potatoes.
3. Skyr parfait: 1 cup Skyr, ¼ cup low-sugar granola, berries, 1 tbsp chia.

Lunch

1. Grain bowl: 6 oz chicken, ¾ cup rice/quinoa, big veg, tahini-lemon.
2. Sushi bowl: 6 oz salmon/tuna, ¾ cup rice, edamame, seaweed salad, avocado, tamari.
3. Lentil & feta salad: 1 cup lentils, arugula, peppers, olives, feta (DF: skip), EVOO.

Dinner

1. Sheet-pan: 6-8 oz chicken thighs, roasted sweet potato (¾ cup), Brussels sprouts.
2. Turkey bolognese: 8 oz turkey over chickpea or GF pasta; arugula salad.
3. Tofu curry: 8 oz tofu, mixed veg, light coconut milk, ¾ cup jasmine rice (parboiled if possible).

Restrictions: Handle as above.

Goal: Body recomposition

Breakfast

1. Pre-train smoothie: whey (30 g), banana, oats (¼ cup), spinach, milk of choice.
2. Egg + toast: 3 eggs, 2 slices sourdough/GF, fruit.
3. Cottage bowl: 1 cup cottage cheese (DF alt), pineapple, honey drizzle, granola sprinkle.

Lunch

1. Burrito bowl: 6-8 oz steak/chicken, 1 cup rice/beans, fajita veg, salsa, avocado.
2. Poke bowl: double fish (8-10 oz), 1 cup rice, seaweed/veg, tamari.
3. Sourdough turkey melt: 8 oz turkey, cheese (DF skip), side salad + fruit.

Dinner

1. Pasta + protein: 3-4 oz dry pasta, 6-8 oz ground bison/turkey, marinara, parmesan (DF skip), side greens.
2. Teriyaki salmon: 8 oz, 1 cup rice, bok choy; use low-sugar sauce.
3. Bean & tofu chili: tofu + 1 cup beans, peppers/onions; cornbread or rice.

Restrictions: Handle as above.

Goal: Cognitive wellness and energy stability

Breakfast

1. Olive-oil eggs (2-3) + smoked salmon, tomatoes, arugula.
2. Yogurt (plain full-fat or Skyr) + berries, walnuts, cinnamon.
3. Chia pudding (chia + almond milk overnight), berries, hemp hearts.

Lunch

1. Sardine-EVOO salad: greens, sardines, olives, capers, lemon.
2. Quinoa-chickpea tabbouleh, cucumbers, parsley, EVOO; add grilled shrimp/chicken.
3. Lentil soup + Greek side salad with 4-6 oz chicken.

Dinner

1. Grilled fish (6-8 oz), ratatouille veg, farro (½-¾ cup).
2. Chicken souvlaki, tzatziki (DF alt), Greek salad, small pita (GF as needed).
3. Mushroom/veg stew over polenta; side arugula with EVOO.

Restrictions: Handle as above.

Goal: Gut repair

Breakfast

1. Bone broth protein smoothie - Bone broth protein powder, spinach (lightly steamed), blueberries, MCT oil, unsweetened almond milk.
2. Soft scramble - 2 whole eggs + 3 egg whites cooked in ghee, zucchini ribbons, fresh herbs. Side: ½ avocado.
3. Collagen chia pudding - Chia seeds soaked overnight in coconut milk, collagen peptides stirred in, topped with cooked apple/cinnamon.

Lunch

1. Wild salmon bowl - 6 oz poached salmon, white rice (½ cup), steamed carrots + zucchini, drizzle EVOO.
2. Shredded chicken soup - Slow-cooked chicken thighs, bone broth, carrots, spinach, herbs. Gluten-free cracker optional.
3. Turkey patty plate - 6-8 oz ground turkey patty, roasted butternut squash, sautéed spinach in olive oil.

Dinner

1. White fish + root veg - 6 oz cod or halibut, mashed parsnip + cauliflower, steamed green beans.

2. Slow-braised lamb shank - Small portion, carrots + zucchini, fresh parsley; side of jasmine rice if tolerated.
3. Egg drop soup - Chicken bone broth base, egg ribbons, bok choy, diced soft tofu.

Restrictions: Handle as above.

Goal: Cardiac health and longevity

Breakfast

1. Skyr + berry bowl - 1 cup Icelandic skyr, ½ cup blueberries/raspberries, 1 tbsp flaxseed, drizzle EVOO.
2. Egg + avocado toast - 2 eggs soft-boiled, 1 slice sprouted grain bread, avocado spread, side tomatoes.
3. Oats + walnuts - ½ cup oats, scoop whey protein, 1 tbsp walnuts, cinnamon, drizzle olive oil.

Lunch

1. Mediterranean salad - 6-8 oz grilled salmon, arugula, cucumber, tomato, olives, EVOO + lemon dressing.
2. Lentil + chicken bowl - 1 cup lentils, 6 oz grilled chicken, sautéed kale, tahini drizzle.
3. Sardine plate - Sardines packed in EVOO, steamed broccoli, side quinoa (½ cup), olive oil + lemon.

Dinner

1. Grilled trout - 6-8 oz trout, roasted Brussels sprouts, small baked potato, EVOO drizzle.
2. Turkey + bean chili - Lean ground turkey, black beans, tomatoes, bell peppers, onions; side salad.
3. Bison stir-fry - 6 oz ground bison, bok choy, mushrooms, garlic/ginger, served with ½ cup barley.

Restrictions: Handle as above.

6. Eating out? Use this restaurant script set as needed.

- "I'll do the **grilled [salmon/chicken/ steak]. No glaze**, sauce **on the side. Double vegetables, swap fries for a side salad** with olive oil and lemon. If available, **add a small potato or ½ cup rice.**"
- Sushi: "**Sashimi or poke** with **double fish, half rice**, extra seaweed/veggies, **tamari** not soy."
- Mexican: "**Fajitas** with extra peppers/onions, **no tortillas, guac on the side**; or **burrito bowl** with half rice, double protein, salsa."
- Breakfast meeting: "**3 eggs**, side fruit, **skip the white-bread toast** (or sub for 1 slice gluten-free or whole grain), add **bacon or smoked salmon.**"

7. Manage, improve, and optimize every **two weeks.**

Follow these two-week adjustment rules (use scale weight, waist circumference, continuous glucose monitoring if applicable, and energy levels).

- **If avg CGM peak >160 mg/dL → cut 25-50 g carbs/day** or move most carbs to breakfast/lunch/peri-workout; add 10-20 g fiber from veg/chia.

- **If AM energy low → add 10-20 g protein** at breakfast and ensure **20-30 g carbs** if training that morning.

- **If evening hunger → add a 4-5 pm bridge:** 10-15 g protein + fiber (e.g., Greek yogurt + chia, or turkey + apple).

- **If weight loss stalls ≥2 weeks → reduce 100-200 kcal/day** (start with carbs) **or** add **1 × 45-60 min. Zone 2** weekly.

- **If training performance drops → move 40-60 g carbs** to pre/post-workout; consider pausing metformin. around intense sessions.

That's not quite all yet. Consider what else your body may need for optimal performance.

Additional Nutritional Considerations

It's necessary to consider other factors that might further

fine-tune your personal nutritional strategy. For example, if you're under **high stress** or struggling with **poor sleep**, long fasts are unwise. Instead, aim for three to four balanced meals a day and make sure you're getting quality protein at breakfast to stabilize energy and mood.

If you live an **athletic lifestyle**, timing your carbs around workouts can make all the difference. Pair this with proven performance supports like creatine and a smart sodium plan to maintain hydration and recovery. On the other hand, if you've been diagnosed with **insulin resistance**, you'll want to prioritize protein and vegetables first at meals, save starches for last, and add a short post-meal walk to blunt blood sugar spikes. Even something as simple as a splash of vinegar can help improve glucose control.

And it's true; of all things, vinegar does help your body control its glucose level. I specifically recommend **1 tablespoon of apple cider vinegar per day**, diluted in water.[117] Need more reassurance that it's worth remembering and consuming daily? From a 2015 paper in the *Journal of Diabetes Research:*

> Vinegar compared to placebo (1) increased forearm glucose uptake ($p = 0.0357$), (2) decreased plasma glucose ($p = 0.0279$), insulin ($p = 0.0457$), and triglycerides ($p = 0.0439$), and (3) did not change NEFA and glycerol.
>
> *Conclusions.* In DM2 vinegar reduces postprandial hyperglycaemia, hyperinsulinaemia, and hypertriglyceridaemia

without affecting lipolysis. Vinegar's effect on carbohydrate metabolism may be partly accounted for by an increase in glucose uptake, demonstrating an improvement in insulin action in skeletal muscle.[118]

From the same paper:

Postprandially, muscle glucose uptake was increased in the vinegar group compared to placebo (AUC0–300 min[*fo*] 765 ± 87 versus 579 ± 63 μmol/100 mL tissue, in vinegar and placebo group, resp., p = 0.0357)[119]

Continuing on the topic of muscle, for women in **perimenopause** or **menopause**, protein becomes even more critical. Aim for 30-40 grams per meal, pairing it all with resistance training to help counteract age-related muscle loss. Fasting should be approached with caution during this stage since hormonal shifts can make extended fasts more stressful on the body.

From a 2023 paper in *BJOG: An International Journal in Obstetrics and Gynaecology*:

Two interacting mechanisms drive net protein breakdown in menopausal women: (i) enhanced protein breakdown, which is acutely reversible with estrogen replacement and (ii) impaired protein synthesis, arising from anabolic resistance to dietary protein, which occurs in men as well as women and is associated with advancing age, and in the context of delayed healing following certain muscle injuries.[120]

The paper goes on to describe the concept of "**protein leverage**":

> A specific appetite for protein dominates regulation of energy intake in many animals, humans included, when faced with nutritionally imbalanced diets—a phenomenon termed protein leverage. Hence, when protein becomes diluted in the food supply by fats and carbohydrates, more energy is necessarily ingested in attaining the target intake of protein that signals satiety. Conversely, as protein becomes more concentrated in the diet, total energy intake is restricted ... Protein requirements increase at times of anabolic demand (e.g. for growth and reproduction) or enhanced net protein breakdown, as described above for the menopause transition. In these circumstances, achieving a higher protein target without exceeding energy needs requires a change in macronutrient balance towards a higher percent protein diet.[121]

In short, the body wants more protein but can't get it, meaning that you eat as much as possible to satisfy this hunger for protein. If you're not getting enough in your diet, you just eat more until you do. Thanks to the dilution of proteins, this turns out to be a lot, leading to increased rates of obesity.

Also, age matters more than sex with regard to protein intake differences—the youngest and oldest among us need more than the middle. (Infants under 1 month need 2.5 grams of protein per kilogram of body weight, shrinking to 1.8 grams per kg between 1 and 2 months, and shrinking further to 1.4 grams between 2 and 4 months. This shrinks further to 0.8 grams until age 65, where it goes up to 1 gram per kilogram of body weight.[122]) Protein needs are not much different between men and women.[123]

Each life stage brings its own demands, and nutritional strategies must adapt accordingly. The right plan is not one-size-fits-all but tailored to your physiology, your goals, and the realities of your everyday life.

Part of your everyday life, a significant part, in fact, is your partner, your family, or both. **Social modeling** is the idea that we do as those closest to us do. This is why sharing a nutrition goal with your partner can have a positive . . . or negative . . . impact. So I don't mean you tell those closest to you your goal, I mean you share it, as in, you both or all have the same goal. Besides the obvious risk of sabotage (e.g., "I made these high-sugar cookies for you; why won't you eat them all? Don't you love me?"), the stress of doubled food preparation is not what you need right now. It takes time to make a meal; it takes as much as twice the time to make two separate meals—one for you, one for the unaligned family. And if you're preparing one meal for yourself but multiple servings of another for multiple family members, that's just not going to work long term.

Nutrition is more than what you put in your mouth; it's your relationship with food. It's complex, personal, intimate, and social. Clinically-precise approaches do not work for long, as do those in which those closest to you are working against you. As with anything health-related, I advise practicality and sustainability . . . which is why I would be remiss to skip a critical set of concerns most people have around their nutrition. We'll grant them the significance due them with their own section.

Cooking and Calorie Counting: Low-Tech Challenge, High-Tech Solution

In the *Run Your Numbers* step earlier in this chapter, I wrote of the mathematical formula to determine how many calories you should be consuming. It then makes sense to assume that you are indeed counting the calories you intake. Yes, that's correct. You should indeed by doing so. It then stands to reason that the more ingredients go into each and every meal, the more calorie-counting you must do. Yes, which is generally unsustainable. Where many people generally struggle with food is cooking. It's a lost art, and most don't have time to keep it up, as the frozen meals section at all supermarkets can attest. And that's not to forget snacking, which has its own issue with high calorie density.

The easiest hack I've found around all of this is to simply use your favorite AI chatbot to advise you on preparing the quickest meal the fastest way and breaking down your daily diet into caloric portions so that you have simple instructions to follow with few ingredients to remember and manage and a virtual guarantee that you will not exceed your target caloric intake.

Perhaps you want to prepare a ground beef-based meal, and you have only twenty minutes before your next thing in the evening. What spices do you have in the pantry? Vegetables in the fridge? Use speech-to-text with your favorite AI tool, tell it your caloric limit, time availability, and ingredients. In literally seconds, you will have an output with preparation time and simple instructions that is better than just about any cookbook you can buy.

Instead of making your life routine revolve around food prep and calorie-counting, leverage AI a little so your food prep and caloric intake revolve around your routine. This is sustainable.

Shifting topics a bit, the principle of sustainability covers other nutrition aspects, including how you choose to (or not to) supplement. Let's see that next.

Supplemental Content about Supplements for Midlife and Beyond

When people ask me, "Are there supplements or vitamins that pretty much everybody in their fifties and beyond should be taking?" my answer is yes . . . but with caveats.

A few staples come to mind right away: **omega-3s**, **vitamin D**, **magnesium**, **creatine**, and a quality whole-food **multivitamin**. That's my own personal stack, and it's also what I often talk through with patients. Beyond those basics, there are targeted options depending on someone's needs.

For example, **berberine** is excellent for metabolic instability—it's essentially on par with metformin, our first-line drug against diabetes. From a July 2025 study in *Frontiers in Pharmacology*:

> [Berberine] exerts its effects through the activation of AMP-activated protein kinase, enhancing glucose uptake in peripheral tissues, promoting lipid metabolism, and influencing fasting plasma glucose (FPG) and TG levels. Additionally, berberine reduces reactive oxygen species production and increases antioxidant enzyme activity, thereby mitigating oxidative stress that contributes to hyperglycemia. Berberine has also been shown to increase HDL-C levels, exhibiting lipid-modulating properties.[124]

Nattokinase, derived from fermented soy, is another; it acts as a fibrinolytic, breaking down blood clots, which are the leading cause of heart attacks and strokes. Some even hypothesize that nattokinase helps explain Japan's remarkable life expectancy. A February 2017 study in the *International Journal of Molecular Sciences* tells us the exact process for this, explaining:

> [Nattokinase] can break down blood clots by directly hydrolyzing fibrin and

plasmin substrate, converts endogenous prourokinase to urokinase (uPA), degrades PAI-1 (plasminogen activator inhibitor-1), and increases tissue plasminogen activator (t-PA) which supports fibrinolytic activity.[125]

Nattokinase has worked wonders in animal models. From the paper:

> When dogs were orally administered four NK capsules (2000 FU/capsule), chemically-induced thrombi in the major leg vein were completely dissolved within five hours and normal blood flood was restored. A rat model of thrombosis in the common carotid artery also demonstrated that NK-treated rats recovered 62% of arterial blood flow. NK exhibited considerably stronger thrombolytic activity than the fibrinogenolytic and fibrinolytic enzymes, plasmin, or elastase; which restored 15% and 0% of blood blow [sic] in the rat carotid artery, respectively.[126]

Nattokinase must not be ignored. But of course there are caveats. Nattokinase is inadvisable if you're on blood thinners; berberine can dangerously lower blood sugar if you're already on insulin or metformin.

On the hormonal side, for men, I'll sometimes layer on **boron, shilajit, tongkat ali**, or **ashwagandha**—all of which have been studied as testosterone boosters. But in my experience, it's about a coin flip. Maybe half the time, someone sees a real rise in testosterone while also working out more, putting on muscle, having more sex—all other lifestyle factors that influence hormones. So if you're trying to go from 300 to 900, supplements alone aren't going to get you there.

For women, especially those with estrogen dominance—say PCOS or menopausal transitions—we'll often use **curcumin, vitamin B complex**, and **zinc**. Two other big ones are **DIM** (diindolylmethane) and **calcium D-glucarate**, which help tamp down excess estrogen. These can also be useful for men on TRT, since testosterone therapy can raise estrogen as well. For bone health, **calcium** paired with **vitamins D3** and **K2** are critical, especially to prevent osteopenia.

Then there are the heart-protective and anti-inflammatory supplements: **CoQ10, quercetin**, and **methylated B vitamins** to reduce homocysteine levels. All of these have good mechanistic support, and we use them often.

And finally, **fiber**, not often thought of as a supplement, ought to be treated as such. Full-fiber foods like legumes with their plant-based protein and iron content are my preference. But odds are, you're among the 95 percent of Americans with insufficient dietary fiber intake.[127] If beans disagree with you—and they do for many, for many reasons—it makes sense to consider fiber a supplement. Psyllium husk, inulin, or partially hydrolyzed guar gum can be a simple way to bridge that gap.[128, 129, 130] Adequate fiber supports gut health by feeding beneficial bacteria, improves stool regularity, and helps regulate blood sugar by slowing carbohydrate absorption.[131, 132, 133] It also promotes satiety, which can aid weight management, and supports cardiovascular health by lowering LDL cholesterol. Per a 2024 study in *Frontiers in Nutrition*:

> . . . [B]oth soluble and insoluble fibers play significant roles in various bodily functions. One key effect of fiber consumption is the enhancement of gastric distension, which occurs when the stomach expands as it fills with food. This process triggers the release of certain hormones from the gut that promote a sense of fullness, known as satiety. Consequently, individuals often find themselves eating less overall. Adopting a diet abundant in fiber not only helps to regulate appetite but also encourages healthier eating habits over time. As people consume less food due to increased feelings of fullness, they are likely to experience weight loss. This reduction in body weight can have profound effects on metabolic health, including better regulation of glucose levels.[134]

In that same paper:

> Dietary fiber is crucial for having a healthy diet for the cardiovascular system. Fiber-rich diets incorporation within the daily meals, can significantly improve overall well-being and heart health . . . Soluble fiber can bind to the bile acids within the digestive tract,

extract them and lowers the cholesterol level in the blood. Studies have proved that the intake of soluble fiber can significantly reduce LDL as an important risk factor for coronary artery disease.

While whole-food sources of fiber remain ideal, supplementation can be a safe, effective tool for people struggling to consistently reach their daily fiber needs. Now, I do need to be clear: Some people *do* overdo it. I've had patients come in with literal bags of supplements, easily fifty different products. Quality control is a huge issue, too. A 2022 study in the *Journal of the American Medical Association* (JAMA) on Amazon-sold supplements found that about half didn't actually contain the amount of the active ingredient on the label:

> This case series study analyzed 30 dietary supplement products purchased from Amazon.com with claims related to immune health. Seventeen of 30 products had inaccurate labels; 13 were misbranded, and 9 had additional components detected but not claimed on the label.[135]

That's why third-party certification, such as the USP Verified Mark or NSF Certified for Sport, are non-negotiable.[136, 137] Where you buy your supplements matters almost as much as which ones you take. And in alphabetically-ordered summary format now, the ones I do suggest are as follows; this is not a shopping list but rather a "these might help you" set of suggestions that are worth looking into as time and budget allow:

- Ashwagandha
- Berberine
- Boron
- Calcium
- Calcium D-glucarate
- CoQ10
- Creatine
- Curcumin
- DIM (diindolylmethane)
- Fiber
- Magnesium
- Methylated B vitamins
- Nattokinase
- Omega-3s
- Quercetin
- Shilajit
- Tongkat ali
- Vitamin. B complex
- Vitamin. D and K2
- Whole-food multivitamin
- Zinc

Finally, I wish we had better trials on many of these. Pharmaceutical drugs get rigorous, large-scale studies. Supplements rarely do, partly because there's no financial incentive. According to the FDA itself, "The FDA does NOT have the authority to approve dietary supplements for safety and effectiveness, or to approve their labeling, before the supplements are sold to the public."[138] Drugs can be patented due to their unique chemical makeup, while supplements are often unpatentable and thus not worth the considerable expense of a clinical trial.[139] The NIH has spent $100 billion between 2010 and 2016 studying pharmaceuticals while spending only $2.4 billion since 1999 studying vitamins and minerals (which cannot be patented.)[140, 141] I would love to see more innovative, crowdfunded approaches to studying naturally occurring compounds with the same rigor as pharma. Until then, I practice with the best evidence we have, my own clinical experience, and careful, individualized guidance for each patient. And that worked for Samantha and Daniel—and can for you, too.

Samantha and Daniel's Stories, Continued

The turning point for Samantha came when we at Velocity encouraged her to stop intermittent fasting. Instead, under the guidance of our director of female optimization, she tried the "bean diet" for menopause symptoms. This approach had already worked well for many others—and for Samantha, it helped stabilize her mood, too. She continued her wellness influencer activities but shifted her focus away from strict diets and nutrition optimization. Instead, she leaned more into lifestyle "hacks" like blue light blocking, red light therapy, and cold plunges. This may not make sense as a success anecdote at first for nutrition, but understand what her de-emphasis meant—*Samantha got it right.* The fact that she didn't have to worry about food anymore . . . there's a win.

Daniel also did what he had to do also, and it worked. All of it. This chapter you've just read. The goal, the system, the food, the work. He did it. And he lost all the unnecessary visceral fat, started to get his athletic body back, was able to move more with his kids and family, and felt better about his legacy—the best he'd felt in years.

Samantha and Daniel never met. One was entering menopause; the other, fatherhood. One had too many health experiments; the other, none. Yet both were at a fork in the road where nutrition made the difference between long decline ahead and an imminent renewal.

They had both employed similar, not "fad diets," but popular techniques. They were swimming in all these data and patterns that weren't bespoke to them, which is exactly what they both needed. And that's the point—nutrition isn't about doing what's popular, it's about doing what's personal.

For Samantha, that meant letting go of the yo-yo trends and simplifying to food that stabilized her hormones and her energy. For Daniel, it meant harnessing tools—yes, even some experimental ones—to rebuild his metabolism and reestablish the confidence of his youth.

The right system works when you work the system. That said, nutrition is only one major component for lasting mid-fifties health transformation. I'll put it this way: Nutrition is fuel; exercise is output. Pair the wrong exercise with the wrong fuel, and the whole system sputters. Pair them correctly, and you build a body that runs like a well-tuned engine. Basically, the more you move, the more you need. Just like a standard car, you don't put the same amount of gas in the tank for a quick trip around the block as you do for a cross-country drive. Your activity level determines your nutritional needs, and if they're mismatched, you'll either run out of fuel—or stall under the weight of unused calories.

Nutrition is subjective and highly individual. What works for one person at midlife may backfire for another, depending on genetics, hormones, and lifestyle. Exercise, on the other hand, is more objective. The body responds in clear, measurable ways to training. Muscles grow, fat shrinks, endurance improves, and blood markers shift. You can see it, track it, test it.

And that's exactly why the next step in your transformation is movement. Nutrition gives you clarity; exercise, certainty. Together, they form the inseparable pair that makes high performance in midlife not simply possible but predictable.

CHAPTER 5
Amplify Physical Fitness

James was a classic founder-turned-CFO, the kind of executive who'd built his company from scratch. He was burning the candle on both ends—burning through work, burning through family responsibilities—and the burn was beginning to hurt badly. He came into Velocity complaining of sluggishness, low energy, and feeling "not himself," but there was no formal diagnosis. He hadn't seen a doctor in years.

Now, that's not unusual for guys like James. No one had told him something was "wrong." He didn't have diabetes, didn't have heart disease, didn't even have high cholesterol flagged on a routine panel. What he did have was the creeping sense he was underperforming in every area of his life. His work wasn't as sharp. His body wasn't as responsive. His wit wasn't as quick. And he wanted to know why.

Within three months of testing, we uncovered three critical issues. First, low muscle mass. On his DEXA scan, James's appendicular lean mass index (ALMI)—the measure of functional muscle in the limbs, adjusted for age and sex—was in the 25th percentile. Not the 75th. Not even the 50th. The 25th percentile. Muscle mass is what we call a glucose sink; it's a great place for blood glucose to get stored. The more muscle you have, the less insulin-resistant you are—the more insulin-sensitive you are, in other words. ALMI predicts whether you'll have the muscle strength to stay functionally independent into older age. Without enough, you're more likely to fall, break a bone, spiral downward, and worse. In summary, James's low ALMI was a red flag. But not the only one.

James's lipoprotein insulin resistance (LPIR) score came back elevated. Most people haven't heard of LPIR. It's an advanced biomarker more predictive of downstream development of diabetes than even a hemoglobin A1c or fasting glucose. His metabolism was indeed quietly sliding toward diabetes.

We also ran a sleep study because James complained of poor sleep and fatigue. Sure enough, he tested positive for moderate sleep apnea. He didn't have the classic signs—he wasn't a loud snorer, and he didn't wake up gasping—but he had a thick neck with adipose tissue compressing his airway. That's enough to rob you of deep sleep and oxygen all night long.

James figured his Peloton rides and occasional swims were "enough." Like low-level cardio equaled health. But cardio alone wasn't fixing the real issues. His body composition was out of balance—muscle mass was too low, which meant (pretty much) that glucose had nowhere to go. His sleep was fragmented; recovery never really happened. His metabolism was stuck in insulin resistance, so his body was primed for fat-storing, not fat-burning.

The writing was on James's wall. His father had

suffered a hip fracture in his seventies. The injury itself wasn't fatal, but what followed was. Within five years, his father was gone. He didn't want his kids to watch him crumble the same way.

I promised James we would not let that happen. And so we changed his training. No more cardio-only routine. We had him start with resistance bands and bodyweight exercises—movements he admitted he didn't identify with at first. He wasn't a "weights guy." But we built him up gradually to 30-45 minutes of compound lifts two or three times a week.

Over the course of the next six months, his scale-weight only dropped five pounds. But that's *net* pounds. The DEXA scan told the whole story—he lost 18 pounds of fat and gained 13 pounds of muscle. His clothes fit differently. His energy rebounded. And his eventual second sleep study showed his apnea had essentially disappeared.

By focusing on muscle, James reversed his insulin resistance, improved his metabolism, and gave himself back the functional strength to live—and protect—his future.

Now, where James under-trained, Oliver over-hacked. By his early 60s, Oliver had become something of a legend in his circle for trying every shiny new "life-extension" trick on the market. He was the guy with the metformin prescription for longevity, NMN capsules for NAD+ boost, stem-cell infusions for regeneration, and a supplement cabinet that looked like a laboratory.

And yet Oliver got winded climbing stairs. His grip strength was slipping. Despite the hacks, his body wasn't keeping up.

So we ran the advanced tests. You would not believe what we found . . . which is probably why you will. Oliver's VO$_2$ max—the measure of cardiorespiratory fitness, essentially how well your heart, lungs, blood vessels, and cells handle oxygen—was below average for his age. His leg muscle mass had diminished, a classic sign of sarcopenia. His IGF-1 was low, likely from chronic metformin. use.

For all his biohacking, Oliver was missing the fundamentals. Oliver had been trying to hack his way into longevity. But what he ignored was the hard work of building longevity. You can't supplement your way around poor cardiorespiratory capacity. You can't out-hack the need for muscle. You just can't. No number of health expert podcasts listened to on double speed can do what a simple fitness routine will.

So we cut the noise. Oliver paused unnecessary compounds that were lowering his IGF-1, and we set him up with the basics—zone 2 cardio and resistance training.

Zone 2 cardio is the aerobic base training most people ignore. Put simply, it's building your lung capacity so your cells get more efficient. The heart, lungs, and blood vessels are strengthened, and your cells get more efficient at using oxygen.[142] For Oliver, that meant regular sessions where he could "talk but not sing" while moving—brisk walking, cycling, steady-state training, and the like. And resistance training, of course, adds back the muscle mass that makes every system work better—metabolism, hormones, stability, longevity. The heart, lungs, and blood vessels are strengthened, and your cells get more efficient at using oxygen.[143] Ten weeks of resistance training may increase lean weight by 1.4 kg, increase resting metabolic rate by 7 percent, and reduce fat weight by 1.8 kg.[144] Resistance training increases testosterone levels in both men and women, though not as strongly for women.[145] And finally, according to a 2023 study by *PLOS One,* greater muscle mass reduces the risk of all-cause mortality.[146]

Here is the takeaway: **Physical activity is a matter of life and death.**

Now, we also changed up Oliver's supplements so they were additive, not trendy. We supervised NAD+ therapy instead of the biohack-scattershot approach he'd been trying.

Within a year, Oliver's VO₂ max rose 20 percent. His strength returned. Everyday activities—stairs, carrying groceries, even long walks—no longer left him winded.

Oliver still enjoys the cutting edge, but now . . . it just works because all the fundamentals are in place. Let's do the same for you.

• • • •

Exercise is by far the most potent longevity "drug." It not only delays death but prevents cognitive and physical decline better than any other intervention. A 2020 study in the *Journal of Physiotherapy* concludes that:

> Exercise reduces global cognitive decline and lessens behavioural problems in people with mild cognitive impairment or dementia. Its benefits on cognitive function are mainly

due to its effects on working memory. The most pronounced effect on global cognition appears to arise from aerobic exercise at moderate or greater intensity with at least 24 hours of total training time.[147]

Meanwhile, physical activity directly fights the muscle loss that naturally occurs with aging.[148]

High aerobic capacity and muscle strength directly translate to lower mortality risk.[149, 150] That's the functional value—vitality, independence, a life that doesn't shrink as you grow older but expands.

As with nutrition in Chapter 4, it all begins with your goals. If your goal is weight loss, there are exercises tailored to that. If your goal is muscle growth, there are different exercises. If your goal is metabolic health, the approach shifts again.

So let's now pair the goals of Chapter 4 right here with Chapter 5—goals like weight loss to the specific exercises recommended. And to do so, let's cover the **Three Pillars of Fitness**. That will make it all make sense.

The Three Pillars of Fitness . . . Especially After 50

These are the big three. You know about two of them already, **VO₂** and **lean muscle**. The specific exercise plan I recommend for you will be based on a primary template, as it were, that is itself set upon all three pillars. We'll just adjust things based on your goals.

Pillar #1: Balance

The first pillar is one many senior citizens wish they hadn't put off for ten, twenty, or more years: balance. (This covers posture and stability as well, by the way.) One of the most important functions of the nervous and musculoskeletal systems is **proprioception**—your body's ability to sense where it is in space. Specifically, the skin, muscles, and joints are involved in its functioning.[151] It's what keeps you upright and moving in the direction you intend to go.

Before jumping into activities like pickleball or weightlifting, you need to get this right. Too many people skip over the basics, move with poor form, and end up injured. Those injuries can be catastrophic, A little socializing with a racquet, some showing off, and suddenly . . . you acting like you're nineteen again knocks you out of normal activity for one to two months, sometimes with lasting damage. Turning back the clock takes time, ironically.

That's why we start with simple assessments at Velocity, like running the "get up and go" test, or standing with one foot in front of the other for a 10-second balance check. These quick screens show us whether your foundation is solid or whether we need to strengthen it before you move on to more demanding exercise. Either way, we will be rebuilding or strengthening from an already-good place.

Next comes, as you might suspect, VO$_2$ max.

Pillar #2: VO₂ Max

If I had to pick just one metric to predict how long—and how well—you'll live, it's this one.

VO₂ max measures how many milliliters of oxygen your body can use per kilogram of body weight per minute. In plain English . . . that means it tells us how efficiently your heart, lungs, blood vessels, and mitochondria (your cells' power plants) work together to produce energy.

Now, get this: Smokers compared to non-smokers have a 40 percent higher chance of all-cause mortality over the coming year, whereas low VO₂ max puts a person at a *400* percent higher risk compared to one with a higher VO₂ max. From a 2018 study published by the JAMA network:

> The increase in all-cause mortality associated with reduced cardiorespiratory fitness (low vs elite: adjusted HR, 5.04; 95% CI, 4.10-6.20; $P < .001$; below average vs above average: adjusted HR, 1.41; 95% CI, 1.34-1.49; $P < .001$) was comparable to or greater than traditional clinical risk factors (coronary artery disease: adjusted HR, 1.29; 95% CI, 1.24-1.35; $P < .001$; smoking: adjusted HR, 1.41; 95% CI, 1.36-1.46; $P < .001$; diabetes: adjusted HR, 1.40; 95% CI, 1.34-1.46; $P < .001$). In subgroup analysis, the benefit of elite over high performance was present in patients 70 years or older (adjusted HR, 0.71;

95% CI, 0.52-0.98; P = .04) and patients with hypertension (adjusted HR, 0.70; 95% CI, 0.50-0.99; P = .05). Extreme cardiorespiratory fitness (≥2 SDs above the mean for age and sex) was associated with the lowest risk-adjusted all-cause mortality compared with all other performance groups.152

Now, let's bring it back to you and your numbers. The gold-standard way to measure is a lab-based test. You hop on a treadmill, bike, or rower, wear an oxygen mask, and gradually ramp up your effort for 10-20 minutes. The machine tracks how much oxygen you're consuming at different intensities. But if you don't have access to a lab, there are simpler options:

- **Cooper's Test**: Run as far as you can in 12 minutes, then plug your distance into a formula.

Here's how this one works.

Measurement	Formula
Distance in meters	VO_2 max (ml/kg/min) = **(Distance in meters - 504.9) ÷ 44.73**
Distance in kilometers	VO_2 max = **(22.351 × kilometers) - 11.288**
Distance in miles	VO_2 max = **(35.97 × miles) - 11.29**

Run the numbers:

1. Run as far as you can in 12 minutes on a flat

course (e.g., track or treadmill).

2. Measure the total distance you covered.

3. Pick the formula that matches your unit of measure (meters, km, or miles).

4. Plug your distance into the formula to estimate VO_2 max.

That's not the only simple test. Next up, we have:

- **1.5-Mile Run Test**: Run it as fast as possible and calculate your VO_2 max from your time.

Source / Type	Formula
General (both sexes)	VO_2 max = **88.02 - (0.0753 × body weight in pounds) - (2.767 × run time in minutes)**
Another version (more complex)	VO_2 max = **65.404 + (7.707 × [sex]) - (0.159 × body weight in kg) - (0.843 × run time in minutes)**

In the second formula, "sex" is coded (i.e., 1 for male, 0 for female) depending on the source.

- "Run time in minutes" should include fractional minutes (e.g. 10 min. 30 sec = 10.5 min).

Run the numbers:

1. Run **1.5 miles** as fast as possible, ideally on a track or treadmill.

2. Record your time in minutes (decimal format is best).
3. Note your body weight (in pounds or kilograms depending on the formula).
4. Plug the numbers into your chosen formula.

Here's a breakdown of VO₂ max percentiles by age and sex, based mainly on the **Cooper Institute / Garmin. standard ratings**, with "Superior," "Excellent," etc. defined.[153] Use this to see how your VO₂ max stacks up.

Cooper's Test / VO₂ Max Percentile Breakdown by Age & Sex

We want Velocity patients in at least the 75th percentile or higher. VO₂ max declines about 10 percent per decade after midlife, even if you stay active. If your VO₂ max is 30 at age 50, by the time you're 70 it could drop to the low 20s—meaning you'd be winded climbing one flight of stairs or walking a single city block. But if you want to hike mountains with your grandkids at 75, you'd better be pushing for the 90th percentile now.

Your two best means to **improve** are as follows:

- **Zone 2 Training**: This is moderate cardio at 60-70 percent of your maximum heart rate (rough formula: 220 minus your age). At this intensity, you're breathing harder, maybe even sweating, but you can still talk in full sentences. Aim for at least 3 hours per week, split however you like—two long rides, six 30-minute sessions, whatever fits your life.

- **High-Intensity Interval Training (HIIT):**

Short bursts at 90 percent of your max heart rate, followed by rest. For example, the "Norwegian 4x4" protocol—four minutes hard, four minutes easy, repeat four times. Sprint intervals (like 50-100 meter dashes, warmed up properly) work too. Even 20-30 minutes a couple times per week makes a huge difference. Don't worry about remembering these now; we'll return to specifics in the actual exercise template and its tweaks.

This January 2019 paper from the *International Journal of Exercise Science* makes clear the benefits that Zone 2 training brings. While this paper does not show a direct increase in VO_2 max from Zone 2 training, it does show an increase in oxygen uptake at the metabolic threshold, or what's called $VO_2\theta$:

> The most important finding of this study is the significantly greater increases in $VO_2\theta$ that occurred in triathletes who spent more than 20% of training time in Zone 2 (between $VO_2\theta$ and $V_E\theta$) compared to those who spent greater than 80% of training time in Zone 1 (below $VO_2\theta$). While on average all participants saw improvement in this measure, athletes in the High group more than doubled their increase in $VO_2\theta$ compared to the Low group ... While VO_{2max} is arguably the most common measure of aerobic capacity, some evidence suggests that $VO_2\theta$ may be comparable or superior.[154]

To get improvements in VO$_2$ max, it also takes HIIT. According to a PLOS ONE study:

> ... [I]nterval training produces improvements in VO$_2$max slightly greater than those typically reported with what might be described as adult fitness based continuous training even though many of the studies were of short duration with limited training sessions per week . . . [L]onger intervals combined with high intensity continuous training can generate marked increases in VO$_2$max in almost all relatively young adults.[155]

Zone 2 builds your aerobic foundation; HIIT pushes your ceiling higher. Together, they can raise your VO$_2$ max, extend your healthspan, and give you the stamina to live the life you actually want, one not limited by fatigue. Or by weakness. And that's what we'll return to next: muscle.

Pillar #3: Lean Muscle

As people age, one of their biggest fears isn't running out of money or even facing disease. It's losing independence. Like being able to bathe yourself, shop for groceries, carry your bags, or simply get up out of a chair without help. The main culprit that robs older adults of these abilities is **sarcopenia**, or age-related muscle loss. We lose about 10 percent of our muscle mass every decade, even if we stay active. In fact, it is worse. According to a January 2019 study in featured *Physiological Reviews,* age-related declines in muscle mass are exponential, not linear.[156]

This makes keeping active an imperative.

Now, most older adults aren't thinking, *I want to run an Ironman in my seventies.* It's more like, *I want to keep doing normal things on my own.* Resistance training is the antidote.

Remember body composition? That's more than fat—or just muscle. MRIs are technically more accurate than a DEXA scan to tell you this, but they're far more expensive and rarely used just for this purpose, so DEXA it is. These give us three critical markers:

- **Subcutaneous fat** - the fat under your skin that can be used for energy.

- **Visceral fat** - fat that wraps around organs, is metabolically active, inflammatory, and highly dangerous.

- **Appendicular Lean Mass Index (ALMI)** - a sex- and age-matched measure of muscle mass in your arms and legs.

Remember, that last one gives us a clearer picture of strength and functional capacity than just looking at overall "lean mass," which includes organs. We're going to need it. Our strength target is clear and obvious—keep visceral fat low, subcutaneous fat controlled, and ALMI in a healthy percentile range.

Do all this, and you'll have **grip strength**. Let's talk about it.

Grip strength has become a standard marker in aging studies. It predicts functional independence because it's tied to practical outcomes. Per *Clinical Interventions in Aging* in 2019:

> . . . [G]rip strength is largely consistent as an explanator of concurrent overall strength, upper limb function, bone mineral density, fractures, falls, malnutrition, cognitive impairment, depression, sleep problems, diabetes, multimorbidity, and quality of life . . . [There is also evidence] for a predictive link between grip strength and all-cause and disease-specific mortality, future function, bone mineral density, fractures, cognition and depression, and problems associated with hospitalization. Consequently, the routine use of grip strength can be recommended as a stand-alone measurement or as a component of a small battery of measurements for identifying older adults at risk of poor health status.[157]

For example, if you stumble and reach for a railing, strong grip strength can mean the difference between catching yourself or suffering a hip fracture. And since hip fractures after age 65 carry a startlingly low five-year survival rate, this one measure matters. A 2022 study in the journal *Cureus* investigated 818 elderly hip fracture highlights this mortality rate:

Age Group	Sex	Superior (≈95th percentile)	Excellent (≈80th percentile)	Good (≈60th percentile)	Fair (≈40th percentile)	Poor / Below Average (<40th percentile)
30-39	Male	≥ 54.0	~48.3	~44.0	~40.5	< 40.5
30-39	Female	≥ 47.4	~42.4	~37.8	~34.4	< 34.4
40-49	Male	≥ 52.5	~46.4	~42.4	~38.5	< 38.5
40-49	Female	≥ 45.3	~39.7	~36.3	~33.0	< 33.0
50-59	Male	≥ 48.9	~43.4	~39.2	~35.6	< 35.6
50-59	Female	≥ 41.1	~36.7	~33.0	~30.1	< 30.1
60-69	Male	≥ 45.7	~39.5	~35.5	~32.3	< 32.3
60-69	Female	≥ 37.8	~33.0	~30.0	~27.5	< 27.5
70-79	Male	≥ 42.1	~36.7	~32.3	~29.4	< 29.4
70-79	Female	≥ 36.7	~30.9	~28.1	~25.9	< 25.9

The survival rate for the entire group at one year was 73.7%; at two years, 62.7%; at five years, 38.6%; and at 10 years,13.7%. The median length of survival was 3.42 years, decreasing by age: for the 65-69 cohort, median survival was 8.18 years, whereas, for those 90 and above, median survival was 1.75 years.[158]

A 2020 study in *Acta Orthopaedica et Traumatologica Turcica,* analyzing 51 men and 41 women, found similar results:

The mortality rate was 18.5% (17 patients) after the first-year follow-up and 25% (23 patients) after the second year. The mortality risk after hip fracture was found to be 11.7 times greater than the similar age group population in the third year. In addition, there was a significant relationship between a low (dependent) preoperative ADL score, advanced age (>80 years), male gender, high ASA score and poor ability to walk (unable to walk), and first- and second-year mortalities (p<0.05).[159]

That said, grip strength isn't a picture-perfect measure. It's often used because it's easy to test in research studies—not because it's the best proxy for overall muscle.[160] Someone might have excellent grip strength from years as a plumber or mechanic, for example, but still be metabolically unhealthy and low in overall muscle mass. That's why when we do grip testing at Velocity, we pair it with more comprehensive tools . . . like that DEXA scan. We have to look beyond the hands, wrists, and forearms. Grip strength is a bit of a misnomer because all muscles are connected one way or another with all other muscles. We want that whole body built up and maintained through resistance training. That doesn't always mean barbells and heavy weights now. Bodyweight training, resistance bands, and simple movements done consistently to muscle fatigue can all stimulate growth and protect independence. So, now that you understand the Big Three, we're going to personalize your workouts for the week based on your goals (from Chapter 4).

4 Steps to Your Workout Plan

Remember, our three pillars are balance (together with stability and posture), VO$_2$ max (which is to say, cardiovascular capacity), and lean muscle mass. Here are four steps to find how you, specifically, can build your own workouts on top of the three pillars.

Step 1: Choose Your Primary Exercise Objective

Like the nutrition goals, you must pick one primary goal to shape your routine:

Goal	Focus
Fat loss	Energy deficit, metabolic conditioning, preserve lean mass.
Metabolic rehabilitation	Reverse insulin resistance, increase mitochondrial biogenesis, Zone 2 bias.
Body recomposition	Progressive overload, hypertrophy training, maximize protein utilization.
Cognitive wellness and energy stability	Anti-inflammatory movement, rhythm, breathwork, HRV support.
Gut repair	Stress relief, focused movement, strength training, breathwork
Cardiac health and longevity	Lactate threshold, Zone 5 intervals, cardiac reserve.

Got it? Good! On to the next.

Step 2: Know the Basic Exercise Template (3-6 Days/Week)

Every patient should begin here before layering their goal-specific programming.

Base Weekly Structure

Day	Type	Details
Mon	**Strength A (Push/ Lower)**	Squat, lunge, overhead press, core stability
Tue	**Zone 2 Cardio**	45-60 min. steady-state (130-150 bpm)
Wed	**Mobility + Balance**	Yoga, functional range conditioning, unilateral work
Thu	**Strength B (Pull/ Upper)**	Deadlift, row, pull-up, horizontal push
Fri	**Zone 2 + Sprint Intervals**	30 min. base + 6x30s sprints
Sat	**Optional**: Recovery walk, hike, swim	
Sun	Rest	Parasympathetic day: sauna, stretching, breathwork

Step 3: Customize by Primary Goal

Below are **complete sample routines**, each goal-specific and mapped to the standard Velocity template.

Fat Loss Protocol

- **Objective:** Maximize caloric output and metabolic flexibility while preserving lean mass.

- **Frequency:** 5-6x/week (low intensity + resistance + metabolic conditioning)

- **Cardio Focus:** High NEAT, 2-3x/week Zone 2, 1 HIIT circuit/week

Weekly Plan

Day	Type	Details
Mon	Strength A	3 sets of 10-12 reps, minimal rest, supersets for metabolic demand
Tue	Zone 2 Cardio	60 min. incline walk (treadmill, ruck, elliptical)
Wed	HIIT Circuit	5 rounds: Airbike (30s), KB swings, burpees, rest
Thu	Strength B	3 sets of 8-12 tempo rows, RDLs, push-ups, planks
Fri	Zone 2 + Sprint	30 min. base + 6 x 30s sprints w/ 90s rest
Sat	Long Walk / Ruck	90+ min. outdoor movement
Sun	Rest / Sauna / Breathwork	

Metabolic Rehab Protocol

- **Objective:** Improve mitochondrial function and insulin sensitivity.

- **Frequency:** 4-5x/week, low-to-moderate intensity

- **Cardio Focus:** Heavy Zone 2 emphasis (80% of cardio sessions)

Weekly Plan

Day	Type	Details
Mon	Zone 2 Cardio	45 min. brisk walk or cycling at 135-145 bpm
Tue	Stability + Resistance	3 sets of 8-12 single-leg RDLs, bird dogs, goblet squats
Wed	Rest or Gentle Mobility	Yoga, breathing drills
Thu	Strength (Full Body)	Compound lifts at moderate intensity
Fri	Zone 2 + Sprints	30 min. base, 3x20s fast intervals
Sat	Long Slow Walk	60-90 min. with heart rate control
Sun	Rest	

Body Recomposition Protocol

- **Objective:** Add lean mass and strength with optimized recovery.

- **Frequency:** 4-5x/week training, 2x/week cardio

- **Progression:** Linear overload, deload every 6-8 weeks

Weekly Plan

Day	Type	Details
Mon	Upper Push	3 sets of 8-12 bench, OHP, dips, cable flies
Tue	Lower Body	3 sets of 8-12 back squat, RDLs, walking lunges, calves
Wed	Zone 2	45 min. incline walk or PNOE-guided session
Thu	Upper Pull	3 sets of 8-12 weighted pull-ups, DB rows, face pulls
Fri	Glutes + Core	3 sets of 8-12 hip thrusts, hamstring curls, planks
Sat	Optional Cardio / Walk	60 min. walk, nasal breathing
Sun	Rest	

Cognitive Wellness and Energy Stability Protocol

- **Objective:** Support HRV, reduce inflammation, enhance neurogenesis.
- **Focus:** Rhythm, breath, gait, nasal breathing, nature exposure

Weekly Plan

Day	Type	Details
Mon	Walk + Light Flow	60 min. walk, nasal breathing, followed by 15 min. yoga
Tue	Zone 2 (Low Impact)	Bike, row, or water aerobics at 120-135 bpm
Wed	Mobility & Breath	FRC, PRI techniques, 4-7-8 breathing
Thu	Strength Lite	Bodyweight, low eccentric load: TRX, bands
Fri	Zone 2 or Hike	Emphasis on connection to environment
Sat	Leisure Movement	Pickleball, swim, garden
Sun	Optional parasympathetic reset	Sauna, meditation, cold plunge

Gut Repair Protocol

- **Objective:** Support parasympathetic

dominance, improve vagal tone, and avoid excessive cortisol spikes from overtraining.

- **Focus:** Movement, minimum viable strength training, deep breaths

Weekly Plan

Day	Type	Details
Mon	Walking + Core	30-45 min. brisk walk + 3 sets of 10-15 planks, crunches, or leg raises
Tue	Strength (Lower)	3 sets of 8-12 squats, lunges, and deadlifts; 30-40 min. total
Wed	Tai Chi / Yoga	30-60 min. gentle flow or balance-focused session
Thu	Sauna + Mobility	15-20 min. sauna + 15 min. foam rolling or stretching
Fri	Strength (Upper)	3 sets of 8-12 push-ups, rows, presses, and curls; 30-40 min. total
Sat	Nature Walk	45-60 min. walk outdoors at a conversational pace
Sun	Meditation Hike	60-90 min. hike, moderate pace, with mindful breathing

Cardiac Health and Longevity Protocol

- **Objective:** Lower BP, improve HRV, and increase VO$_2$ max.
- **Focus:** Vascular health, aerobic base

Weekly Plan

Day	Type	Details
Mon	Zone 2 + Strength	30-40 min. Zone 2 cardio (60-70% max HR) + 3 sets of compound lifts (squats, deadlifts, presses)
Tue	Long Walk	45-60 min. brisk walk outdoors at a conversational pace
Wed	Strength	3 sets of 8-12 on major muscle groups; focus on progressive overload (push, pull, legs)
Thu	VO_2 Intervals	4x4 min. at ~90% max HR with 4 min. rest between; build VO_2max capacity
Fri	Zone 2 + Core	30-40 min. Zone 2 cardio + 3 sets of core work (planks, leg raises, rotational moves)
Sat	Hike or Swim	60-90 min. steady Zone 2 hike in nature or lap swim for aerobic base
Sun	Breathwork + Sauna	15-20 min. guided breathwork + 15-20 min. sauna for recovery and nervous system reset

Step 4: Apply Overlays and Consider Constraints

As in Chapter 4, there may be additional considerations for your specific health situation that further tweaks your exercise routine.

Medical Constraints

- **Cardiac history → supervised cardio; VO2** max threshold testing
- **Arthritis/Osteo → low-impact resistance bands, aquatic training**
- **Osteoporosis → impact loading (walking, jumps, stair step)**

Hormonal / Age Overlays

- **Menopause → higher resistance training volume to protect bone**
- **Andropause → prioritize intensity over frequency to manage fatigue**
- **Adolescents / Elderly → skill-based movement; balance priority**

Logistics / Lifestyle

- **Travel → Resistance bands + bodyweight protocol**

- **Busy professionals → 3x/week full-body + daily 30-min. walk**
- **Beginners → Start with 3-day split, focus on form, use DEXA for ALMI tracking**

We'll close this section with my paraphrase of a popular Scott Adams quote, a reality-check reframe on fitness from the most influential personal development author of the modern era. And it goes like this, "The best workout is the one you're willing to do."

And now I'll turn to you before we turn back over to James and Oliver.

Which workout are you willing to do? That's the best one for you.

James and Oliver's Stories, Continued

James and Oliver lived very different lives. James under-trained his muscles; Oliver over-hacked his biochemistry. Yet both were missing the same truth: Fundamentals matter most. It's so important for us to measure what matters and to build a program around people that moves the meaningful metrics forward while rationalizing all of the other stuff around the health and wellness space.

For James, that meant recognizing muscle as his best defense against insulin resistance, falls, and frailty. For Oliver, that meant recognizing VO₂ max as a stronger predictor of life expectancy than any pill or injection.

Both had to relearn the basics—build muscle, build lung capacity, then layer on everything else.

The Ultimate Asset

CHAPTER 6
Fortify Mental Resilience

Sarah's case shows how much mental health is shaped not just by mindset, but by biology. By the time she came to us, she had already been handed the "default" solution so many women in midlife are given—another prescription for SSRIs. Symptoms like low energy, brain fog, irritability, mood swings got brushed off as anxiety or depression. Deeper, root-cause questions were not asked. What's happening with her hormones? What about her thyroid? Could her nutrition be at the root of her mental fog and fatigue?

Once we dug into her labs, the real story emerged. Shifting estrogen and progesterone levels from early perimenopause, a subtle thyroid slowdown, and borderline iron deficiency had conspired against her energy, focus, and mood. She wasn't "depressed," she was *suppressed*. And so the plan we built for Sarah touched both the nutrient side of mental health—dietary changes to restore iron, protein, and micronutrients—as well as the practical side. We wrote out a wind-down routine that protected her sleep, supporting thyroid and hormonal balance, and addressing the mental burdens of her lifestyle. We also encouraged Sarah to delegate more at work, practice morning meditation, and protect her bandwidth at home and in the office.

Stress is a whole body experience, and so, too, is the solution to it. And the body, quite obviously, includes the brain. Health of the mind, for Sarah and for you, can be restored with clinical and nutritional interventions, yes. But also, with practical, even conversational ones. With, in a word, **reframes**. That's where you make a deliberate shift from viewing the glass half-empty, to half-full, simply by changing the angle from which you view it.

And many of us need such a reframe for middle age. To show you what I mean, let's compare and contrast the mental health of a thirty-year-old versus a fiftysomething.

A Tale of Two Seasons

Consider: A thirty-year-old often suffers from accidental or unintentional sleep deprivation. Little kids keep them up, their schedule is dictated by family rhythms, and their mental performance suffers. But a fiftysomething loses sleep for a different reason. Not external disruptions . . . internal ones. It's thought-creep. *I'm over the hill. Life is coming at me fast—and it's leaving even faster.* A thirty-year-old still imagines themselves a young adult, with so much to look forward to. But a fifty-year-old looks back and sees themselves closer to the nursing home than their college glory days. And this is the mental picture of midlife, for many—the sense that time is running out, doors are closing, the train has already left the station.

There's a viral video I saw recently which illustrates this poignantly, called "Aging in Perspective"[161] by The McFarlands channel on TikTok. A young man goes about his day when strangers stop him to ask if he needs help picking up some change off the ground, crossing the street, and so on. He brushes them off; why would he need help? But soon comes the startling reveal—this "young" man is actually very old, but in his mind, he is still himself. That's aging. Outwardly, you can try to hide it—Botox, facelifts, hair dye, sports cars, hormone therapy. Inwardly, you may still feel left behind, chasing a train you'll never catch.

And now it's time for your reframe. **There's always another train.** The longer you stay on the tracks mourning the one that left, the more likely you are to get run over by the next. Mental resilience is about getting back to the station, ready to board the opportunities arriving now, eager for what still is coming your way with blessings and bounty.

Over the hill is not under it. For most of human history, the median lifespan was significantly lower than today. From HumanProgress.org:

> Average life expectancy at birth for people hovered at about 30 years for most of human history. The reason was mostly that about one-third of children died before they reached their fifth birthday. Demographers estimate that in 16th-century England, 60 out of 100 children would die before the age of 16. Some

> fortunate people did have long lives, but only 4 percent of the world's population generally lived to be older than 65 years before the 20th century . . . During the past 200 years, global life expectancy has more than doubled, now reaching more than 72 years . . .[162]

And unless you were born into an elite family, your life would be both short and painful—so painful your skeleton would be the marks of acute injuries, improper healing, poor nutrition, and chronic disease for archeologists to discover centuries, even millennia later.[163] In such a world, puberty marked the beginning of middle age. So if you're reading this in your forties, fifties, or sixties, you've already outlived many of your ancestors' expectations. That alone is a gift-reward of civilization.

With that gift come benefits a thirty-year-old doesn't yet have—the wisdom of decades, the clarity of hindsight, the freedom to pursue dreams without the burdens of little kids or the chaos of early adulthood. Your glory days don't have to be behind you; they can begin tomorrow.

Think of the leaders who shape our world—CEOs, governors, founders, generals, senators and congresspeople, heads of NGOs. The sweet spot of peak contribution is not the twenties, it's the fifties and sixties. That's when experience, influence, and wisdom all finally converge. Some wallow in nostalgia for high school. Others lead the world. The difference between middle-aged decline and undying drive is a fortified mindset, one not of dread but of desire.

You don't have to chase the past anymore. The present and the future are coming into the station of your life. Yes, stress will still come. And again, not an existential dread, but the taxing issues of everyday life, like conflicts at work, the burdens at home, the daily grind. And that's OK, because here is where tools matter. Tools to shift your physiology, your thought patterns, your daily anchors. True peak performance is impossible if your emotional architecture is fragile, brittle. Resilience is as important as VO_2 max or lean muscle measures.

That's why I want to give you a three-part mindset-fortifier framework. Think of it as your Mental Health Stack—three practices you can layer together to fortify your mind the way resistance training enmassens muscle.

Your Mental Health Stack

Let's begin.

The Foundation: Baseline Clinical Mental Health

Before you assume your mental health challenges are "just stress" or "just aging," pause. Many people go years, even decades, with undiagnosed conditions dragging down their energy, focus, and mood. The smartest move you can make is to check this box first.

Screen for Hidden Issues

Ask your doctor (or a precision clinic) to run through these baseline tests. We've covered a few of these previously, but they return with renewed importance where your mental health is concerned.

- **Mood and Cognitive Screens**: Questionnaires for depression, anxiety, ADHD, and burnout. These pick up what casual conversations may not.

- **Sleep Studies**: Many adults have undiagnosed sleep apnea or circadian rhythm disorders. These wreck mood and focus more than most realize.

- **Lab Panels**: Look at thyroid, vitamin D, ferritin (iron), B12, and inflammatory markers. Subclinical deficiencies often masquerade as "depression."

- **Advanced Options**: Cognitive testing, heart-rate variability tracking, or cortisol curve tests can reveal stress patterns your bloodwork misses.

These checks give you clarity where previously there may have been confusion. Next . . .

Avoid Default Prescription Peril

Too often, midlife professionals (especially women in perimenopause) are handed SSRIs when they report fatigue, brain fog, or mood swings. While medication has its place, it shouldn't be the first reflex. A meta analysis from the *Journal of the American Medical Association* shows a nearly 20 percent risk reduction of depression just by getting *half* the recommended amount of daily exercise.[164] From that same paper:

> Accumulating an activity volume equivalent to 2.5 hours of brisk walking per week was associated with 25% lower risk of depression, and at half that dose, risk was 18% lower compared with no activity. Only minor additional benefits were observed at higher activity levels.[165]

Following this book, you'll already be doing far, far better than that.

If your thyroid is underactive, if your iron is low, or if your sleep is broken, a pill may not solve the root cause either. Please consider giving your dietary and fitness changes from Chapters 4 and 5 a little time to percolate into your symptoms and notice any changes worth, well, noticing!

Even if we do diagnose a legitimate health condition like depression among Velocity patients, SSRIs or other prescriptions for their specific situation are an unlikely first step for us. Ample data suggest, once again, dietary interventions and exercise as more efficacious than pills in treating in particular mental health conditions that are not (yet) severe.[166, 167, 168, 169] From a 2022 paper:

> Most reviews in severe mental illness, and

depression and anxiety reported conclusions supporting the positive effects of dietary intervention, including positive effects on weight-related or mental health outcomes, and on mental health outcomes, respectively.[170]

From a 2024 BMJ paper:

Compared with active controls (eg, usual care, placebo tablet), moderate reductions in depression were found for walking or jogging (n=1210, κ=51, Hedges' g −0.62, 95% credible interval −0.80 to −0.45), yoga (n=1047, κ=33, g −0.55, −0.73 to −0.36), strength training (n=643, κ=22, g −0.49, −0.69 to −0.29), mixed aerobic exercises (n=1286, κ=51, g −0.43, −0.61 to −0.24), and tai chi or qigong (n=343, κ=12, g −0.42, −0.65 to −0.21). The effects of exercise were proportional to the intensity prescribed.171

Once you've ruled out or addressed previously undiagnosed and/or unaddressed conditions with fitness and food, continue on to non-invasive approaches that retrain both brain and body such as . . .

- **Cognitive Behavioral Therapy (CBT):** The gold standard for reframing negative thought loops and building stress resilience. As stated in the journal *Focus: The Journal of Lifelong Learning in Psychiatry,* CBT is "a first-line, empirically supported intervention for anxiety disorders" and "a family of techniques that are designed to target maladaptive thoughts and behaviors that maintain anxiety over time."[172] Per *Biopsychosocial Medicine,* it "helps individuals to eliminate avoidant and safety-seeking behaviors that prevent self-correction of faulty beliefs, thereby facilitating stress management to reduce stress-related disorders and enhance mental health."[173] CBT "also has been demonstrated to be effective as an adjunctive treatment to medication for serious mental disorders such as bipolar disorder and schizophrenia."[174]

- **Hypnotherapy:** Proven to help with anxiety, and pain by shifting subconscious patterns that fuel stress. A 2023 meta-analysis in *Frontiers in Psychology* found that "[o]ur findings underline the potential of hypnosis to positively impact various mental and somatic treatment outcomes, with the largest effects found in patients experiencing pain, patients undergoing medical procedures, and in populations of children/adolescents."[175] In a 2019 meta-analysis done by the *International Journal of Clinical and Experimental Hypnosis,* people "treated with hypnosis improved more than about 84% of control participants. Hypnosis was more effective in reducing anxiety when combined with other psychological interventions than when used as a stand-alone treatment."[176] It has even been shown to reduce exam anxiety in students and performance anxiety in athletes.[177]

- **Brain Mapping and Neurofeedback**: Neurofeedback has been proven effective in fighting PTSD as well as ADHD.[178], [179] A June 2024 study in the journal *Cerebral Cortex* even states that neurofeedback is somewhat effective in dealing with depression.[180] We partner with Braincode Centers to help us to re-train patients' minds; learn more at www. braincodecenters.com

Your mental health "healthspan" is as critical as your physical one. If your emotional architecture is shaky, you'll struggle no matter how good your diet or workouts are. But if you start by testing, uncovering hidden issues, and applying the safest, most effective therapies first, you give yourself the best chance at clarity, calm, and confidence.

The Structure: Resilience-Building

If baseline testing is about uncovering what's broken, the next entry in the stack is about building what lasts. Mental resilience is like muscle tissue—trainable, adaptable, expandable with the right kinds of stress, called *eustress*.

Such resilience comes from controlled adversity. When you face discomfort on your terms—think a tough conversation, a hard workout, a deliberate digital detox—you are rewiring your nervous system to handle real-world stress with greater calm. This is exposure therapy in its simplest form; your "chill" response can become trained, rather than you just getting triggered.

Failure, reframed as such, can become rehearsal. Each time you put yourself into a tough situation and come out intact, your brain's anterior cingulate cortex (or ACC, the seat of conflict-monitoring, error correction, and discipline) adapts. Over time, you become less rattled by uncertainty, setbacks, or even crisis. A 2021 study in the journal *eNeuro* points out how important the ACC is to managing distress:

> . . . [a]nalysis indicated greater connectivity between the ACC and dorsolateral prefrontal cortex (DLPFC) in subjects who persisted throughout the task, along with greater FC between the ACC and the precentral gyrus in those who quit before its termination. The results shed light on the mechanisms underlying interindividual differences in the ability to handle distress.[181]

Doing hard things has a cumulatively protective effect; it's more than a cold-plunge fad. There is a real, positive, physiological response to doing things we don't want to do. These are micro-stressors, and doing them helps fire up your ACC, build your resiliency, stretch your perseverance, and enliven your tenacity, the very lifeblood of our existence. So engaging in the thing you don't want to do, or avoiding the thing you really want can actually keep your brain young.

The ancient Stoics had an expression for this practice of micro-stressing. Called *askesis*, it is defined as "the disciplined practice of training one's mind and character toward virtue."[182] Voluntary discomfort is key to Stoic practice, because it allows the practitioner to test the limits of what can be endured.[183] Voluntary discomfort can include skipping a meal after you've had a larger portion than usual, taking a cold walk where it's just outside the range of comfortably warm, and imagining the worst-case scenario ("negative visualization") so you are able to hope for the best yet plan for the no-surprises worst in all things. This last example in particular inoculates you against shock when something truly difficult happens. You've been there, done that, in your mind's eye, and you've figured it out.

This leads us to neuroplasticity, which is exactly what all this mental exertion does for you.

Use Your Mind—Or Lose It

Adults who keep challenging themselves maintain sharper memory, better focus, and greater creativity well into later decades. Resilience practices help deter dementia by keeping neural networks flexible. From a 2022 paper in *Psychological Science*:

> The present research found that people with higher levels of well-being can tolerate higher levels of [Alzheimer's Disease and Related Dementias]-related neuropathology without experiencing memory and thinking

impairments (i.e., greater cognitive resilience). Importantly, the association of well-being with cognitive resilience was observed even when analyses accounted for other known cognitive resilience factors and was among the strongest and most consistent associations compared with these other factors. This research suggests that well-being should be a focus of resilience-based prevention models and may be a powerful target of interventions aimed at preventing or delaying the onset of dementia.[184]

Little micro-adversities help you; that is, intentionally doing or saying or thinking things just outside the edge of comfort stack up and make you a little more resilient each time. Each week, you strengthen the architecture of resilience, just as surely as lifting weights builds muscle.

If you don't use it, you lose it.

The Peak: Social Health Optimization

If resilience is the structure of mental health, relationships are the peak. The best data we have on what keeps people alive and thriving isn't a lab result or a supplement stack. It's the people they surround themselves with.

The Harvard Study of Adult Development has tracked men and their families for more than 80 years. Its conclusion is simple and profound—the quality of your relationships at age 50 predicts your health at age

80. Not cholesterol, income, or genetics have such a strict correlation with quality of life.[185] This is backed up by a study on long-married couples that correlates relationship quality with better health outcomes.[186]

Social isolation carries more mortality risk than smoking a pack of cigarettes per day, by the way.[187] Earlier in my career, I worked for a legendary CEO who implemented a "Chief Togetherness Officer" whose job was to systematically build connection with those we served. Executives up and down the chain were gently required to reach out to lonely seniors and simply have conversations with them. Impacts were profound and actually changed outcomes. Even the National Health Service in the UK has a Minister for Loneliness to address this "real and diagnosable scourge."[188]

This means that social health *is* health. Friendships, family ties, and community connections are thus as important as eating well, exercising, and getting quality sleep. Nurture yourself, nurture others. One or two confidants matter more than dozens of casual contacts. Who can you be truly honest with? Treat them like family you love, even if they're merely friends or friendly acquaintances.

Consider tracking your "social nutrition" also. A 2019 paper in the journal *Human Communication Research* states that having a certain amount of social interaction improves your well-being.[189] A 2019 report on this idea by *Psychology Today* notes that alone time is just as important, stating that "[a]fter analyzing swaths of data, the researchers discovered that a blend of everyday interactions that fortify meaningful social networks combined with some 'contented' alone time was linked to higher degrees of life satisfaction and flourishing."[190]

Just as you measure steps or protein intake, notice how many meaningful interactions you have per week or month. If it's close to zero, your mental health is probably starving for true nourishment. And if you're struggling to find friendly connection, be first to offer it. Listening well, managing conflict without escalation, and expressing gratitude keep bonds alive. A likeminded community has long been a go-to environment for such socializing. A small group, faith circle, hobby club, or volunteer organization can anchor you in belonging. Isolation is the silent killer of middle age. Once it gets bad, it gets worse.

It doesn't have to go that way. These tips will help. But I want more than improvement for you; I want transformation. So let me tell you about . . .

The Gratitude Multiplier

One of the most practical ways to strengthen relationships and your own mental well-being— is gratitude. Don't just journal about it (to yourself; that's basically thankfulness-masturbation. No, get a partner. Send it outward. Let love flow and grow, even platonically so.)

Once a day, send a genuine thank-you note, text, or voice memo. It can be small, like thanking a colleague for their effort, or a child for their thoughtfulness. These unexpected signals compound. They strengthen your network, lift others, and give you immeasurable benefits in return, like lower stress hormones, more endorphins, better mood. Turns out these are, in fact, measurable.

Think of the gratitude multiplier as using your brain's reticular activating system for goodness. The more you practice spotting reasons to be thankful, the more your brain will find them. Gratitude turns your attention from what's missing to what's abundant—and abundance is contagious. As it goes out from you, so will it return to you many, many times over.

Tell others what you appreciate about them, and you will appreciate yourself; you may even feel like yourself again, which may not have been the case for a very long time. This was Sarah's experience.

Sarah's Story, Continued

Within months of onboarding with Velocity, Sarah reported feeling "herself again." Not medicated into numbness, not grinding through fatigue, but genuinely clear-headed and steady. It was like she had rolled back the clock ten years.

Part of that transformation came from going deeper than the default. We did *not* give her yet another prescription or suggest she "just try to stress less." We ran in-depth screenings with validated tools to rule out organic causes of disease, mapped her hormone and thyroid function, and then helped her rebuild her structure with "voluntary discomfort." For her, this meant cold showers and hard sprints after yoga—micro-stressful practices of controlled adversity that sharpened her mental edge instead of softening it.

Sarah also committed to one deceptively simple practice: gratitude texts. Every day, she reached out to a family member or friend with a simple note of specific thanks. Those texts sparked conversations she'd been missing, inspired travel she probably wouldn't have otherwise enjoyed, and rebuilt meaningful emotional connection she hadn't yet realized she'd long ago lost. Now, it was back. So, between the clinical, the physical, and the social, Sarah had a fresh, sturdy foundation well-set enough to carry her through her busiest, most stressful days, which, by comparison, really didn't feel all that stressful anymore.

Now, Sarah's journey is more than her own story. It's a reminder that if you've been struggling with similar symptoms, there may be more going on beneath the surface than the quick fix you were offered. Sometimes what weighs on your mind is less about who you are and more about what your body—and brain—needs. We human beings are social animals. We need people to be well. And one of those people . . . is yourself. You count. You matter. And that's why we want you to be your best. There is so much to look forward to.

The Ultimate Asset

CHAPTER 7

Measure What Advanced Diagnostics Matter

That last chapter on mental resilience was the capstone of what we've called the **core four**: **sleep**, **nutrition**, **exercise**, and **mental health**. Each of these areas stands on its own, and you've now seen how critical they are for both longevity and quality of life. But taken together, they add up to something more than the sum of their parts.

Now we're shifting gears. Up to this point, you've had mostly biology-level advice—specific habits, practices, and interventions you can apply in your daily life. In this next phase, we move from the individual to the systemic. From intentional avoidance of both burnout and biohacking . . . to **biomastery**. This is the systems-view of healthspan. It's not just about what you do in isolation, but how you organize, integrate, and sustain the core four across the long arc of your life. Think of it as practical systems advice—strategies for weaving everything together into a durable lifestyle. From beginner to intermediate to now mastery.

To show you what that looks like in practice, let's return to two people you've already met earlier in this book. Their journeys will illustrate what it means not only to improve each pillar but to align them into a system that actually lasts.

• • • •

Fine is a four-letter word.

Brian, that 49-year-old CEO from Oregon, had been told time and again that he was exactly that. His annual physicals never flagged a thing. But behind the normal numbers, his health was quietly abnormal and worsening. When we dug deeper with advanced diagnostics, the truth emerged—his insulin resistance was measurable through an LPIR score (a test most primary care doctors never run), his thyroid panel showed subtle inefficiencies across free T3, free T4, and reverse T3, and his daily cortisol curve revealed stress hormones raging from morning to night. And then a sleep study uncovered moderate apnea he never suspected. He wasn't the classic snorer waking his partner, but his oxygen dipped enough to drain his energy and cloud his days. In military terms, Brian was facing a low-intensity conflict—a battle, yes, but not so kinetic it could be called war and activate the full force of the American sickcare system to fight back.

Brian's turning point came when we at Velocity designed a custom healthspan plan. Instead of accepting his "fine," he learned how each system in his body could be optimized. He shifted his schedule to match his genetics, finding his natural rhythm again. He built back functional muscle mass, rising from the 25th percentile of the all-important ALMI to the 50th percentile. His body composition shifted dramatically—nearly twenty pounds of fat gone, more than a dozen pounds of muscle gained, with little change on the scale but a profound change in how he looked and performed. For the first time in years, he felt like his energy matched the life he was trying to live.

Then recall Eric, 45, who came to us from the opposite end of the spectrum. A competitive athlete, he assumed he was basically invincible for his age. He looked cut, raced hard, and scoffed at the idea of medical oversight. But the scans told another story. A coronary calcium test revealed early arterial plaque, his cholesterol subfractions showed patterns that predict higher risk, and his body was showing signs of overtraining: chronic inflammation, elevated cortisol, and blood sugar creeping upward despite his lean frame. The very training that made him look like a statue was suppressing his testosterone, a common outcome when body fat drops to single digits and the hypothalamus and pituitary go into survival mode. Hardly optimal.

And so we built Eric a recovery-first program—structured deload weeks every six to eight weeks, recalibrated training to include more Zone 1 and Zone 2 cardio, and flexibility work to keep his system balanced. Nutrition was tweaked with strategic timing and supplementation. Slowly, his testosterone rebounded into the healthy 500s and 600s. Even better, his inflammation dropped, his labs normalized, and his body finally started repairing itself between efforts. Within a season, he went from finishing near the podium to actually standing on top of it, winning races he previously couldn't crack. As he later told us, "I didn't know until I went looking. And that was the missing unlock I needed to get that last one percent better. That meant the difference between winning and losing in my line of business."

Comprehensive Executive Health Assessments

The ordinary check-up simply isn't enough if you care about prioritizing longevity. Standard labs and stethoscopes can only take you so far beyond symptoms-of-the-moment; we need precision. Enter advanced diagnostics.

The goal, obviously, is to get the crystalist-clear picture of your current healthspan. By quantifying the systems most responsible for performance, energy, and resilience, you can spot hidden risks years before they manifest as disease. What you can measure, you can manage.

Take the Coronary Artery Calcium (CAC) score. It's one of the simplest, most affordable scans available, yet it can reveal silent heart disease risk long before symptoms appear. A zero score offers powerful reassurance. A higher score, on the other hand, signals that plaque has already formed in your arteries and your risk of heart attack is rising.

For even deeper insight, there's Coronary CT Angiography (CCTA). Unlike the CAC scan, which shows calcified plaques, CCTA can detect so-called "soft plaques"—the unstable buildups that may rupture and block an artery–by directly visualizing the lumen of blood vessels.[191, 192] Some clinics now use AI-driven analysis to characterize plaque morphology and precisely assess cardiovascular risk; as a 2024 study on AI-driven artery imaging said in *Therapeutic Advances in Cardiovascular Disease*, "Several programs have been developed to further develop AI-CCTA. Among programs with FDA approval are Cleerly and HeartFlow which serve as AI-based digital platforms to improve clinician identification of high-risk plaques."[193] This matters because two people with identical cholesterol numbers might have very different realities inside their arteries—one with clean vessels and no urgency to medicate, another with unstable plaque who needs aggressive therapy. The American College of Cardiology warns that "half of healthy patients with normal cholesterol levels have dangerous plaque build-up in their arteries."[194] According to a 2017 study in the *Journal of the American College of Cardiology*:

> Subclinical atherosclerosis (plaque or coronary artery calcification) was present in 49.7% of CVRF [Cardiovascular Risk Factors]-free participants. Together with male sex and age, LDL-C was independently associated with atherosclerosis presence and extent, in both the CVRF-free and CVRF-optimal groups (odds ratio [×10 mg/dl]: 1.14 to 1.18; p < 0.01 for all). Atherosclerosis

presence and extent was also associated in the CVRF-free group with glycosylated hemoglobin levels.

Many CVRF-free middle-aged individuals have atherosclerosis. LDL-C, even at levels currently considered normal, is independently associated with the presence and extent of early systemic atherosclerosis in the absence of major CVRFs. These findings support more effective LDL-C lowering for primordial prevention, even in individuals conventionally considered at optimal risk.[195]

The more you know, the sooner you can act. The sooner you act . . . you get the idea.

As you might expect, there are other tools that give us equally actionable insights. Like the CAC, we've also previously mentioned the DEXA scan, which shows both bone density and body composition to highlight the difference between subcutaneous fat (energy reserve) and visceral fat (the metabolically-dangerous type that wraps your organs). And of course, a VO_2 max test can quantify your cardio-fitness age, one of the single best predictors of longevity. Together, these tests transform vague impressions like "I feel OK" into hard data you can track and improve.

This whole approach to measure-manage is precision, not paranoia (or profit). We're looking for the levers that matter most for prevention and performance. And what you may not know but have probably guessed already . . . diagnostics extend far beyond these. Next, we'll look at advanced blood panels and even genomic and epigenetic testing—two categories of insight that reveal the deeper stories your biology is telling. Let's start with the latter.

Genomic & Epigenetic Testing

There's a saying in medicine: *Genes load the gun; environment pulls the trigger.* Genomics tells us how the gun is loaded—i.e., what risks are built into your DNA—while epigenetics reveals how your lifestyle, choices, and environment determine whether the trigger is ever pulled.

One of the most useful examples is the APOE gene. APOE codes for a protein that helps us metabolize fats in the brain; it is thought that "problems with brain cells' ability to process fats, or lipids, may play a key role in Alzheimer's and related diseases."[196] Most people have the APOE3/3 variant, which carries baseline risk. A 2016 study on this gene in *Current Alzheimer's Research* noted that 50 to 75 percent of their control populations had this variant.[197] But if you inherit a single copy of APOE4 (APOE3/4), your risk of Alzheimer's and dementia increases *4X*; if you inherit two copies (APOE4/4), your risk jumps to roughly *12X* that of the general population.[198] We are not making the correlation-causation mistake in reasoning here. From a September 2021 study in *Science Translational Medicine*:

> The E4 allele of the apolipoprotein E gene (APOE) has been firmly established as a genetic risk factor for many diseases including

cardiovascular diseases and Alzheimer's disease (AD), yet its mechanism of action remains poorly understood.[199]

This "dementia gene" is implicated in other diseases of aging as well. From the study: "The APOE4 genotype is . . . associated with cardiovascular diseases, increases risk for metabolic syndrome, and is linked with decreased lifespan."[200]

This sort of information isn't destiny, fortunately; it's guidance. Knowing you have APOE4 doesn't mean you will develop dementia, but it does mean that controlling blood sugar, exercising consistently, and getting restorative sleep become absolutely essential to quality and quantity of years.

Genetic testing can also guide medical decisions. Roughly half of patients prescribed common drugs like antidepressant SSRIs or blood thinners carry genetic variants that make those medications less effective or ineffective altogether. Thoughts of self-harm, with the occasional tragic follow-through on such thoughts, are a known risk or certain psychoactive medications that genomics would have otherwise said to avoid.[201] *Arteriosclerosis, Thrombosis, and Vascular Biology,* a journal of the American Heart Association, published a 2019 study which found that 30 percent of Americans carry a gene that blocks the action of clopidogrel, a common blood thinner.[202] Among Asians, this jumps to 45 percent, per the same study. Without testing, doctors may prescribe blindly, leading to trial-and-error cycles that cost time, money, and sometimes . .

. lives. But with pharmacogenetic data in hand, care can be targeted from the start and thus prevent unnecessary side effects or failures.

There's more that we find with such comprehensive tests. You may be familiar already with early consumer tests like 23andMe, which analyze single nucleotide polymorphisms (or, SNPs). These are tiny variations correlated with conditions such as Crohn's or celiac disease. Today, more advanced approaches like whole genome sequencing and exome sequencing go deeper, further, faster, better, in my educated opinion. Such tests identify not just correlations but *deterministic* risks—correlation *with* causation, you might say—to provide clarity on which genes are coding for which proteins and thus affecting which aspect of health.

It's worth it. All of it is. Even so, the cost of sequencing has plummeted since the days of the Human Genome Project, which cost $2.4 billion to start, run, and complete.[203] Today, comprehensive testing can be done for a few hundred dollars (though this depends on health insurance coverage).[204] Prenatal screening, for example, can directly assess chromosomal variants such as trisomy 21 (Down syndrome), with a false positive rate of 0.2 percent; this means it's extremely reliable.[205] The technology is improving rapidly and becoming increasingly accessible. It's not just for expecting mothers and the ancestry-curious consumer.

Now, you might be wondering, *If I can get a genetic test for just a few dollars, why do I need expert help?* Because the raw results are hardly enough to tell you what to change, what not to change, and why (either way).

What matters is interpretation; that is, making sense of the findings and translating them into an individualized, evidence-based plan. AI-generated reports can flag risks, but they don't connect those risks to diet, exercise, hormones, or, frankly, life goals. That's the difference between data and wisdom. Companies like Velocity specialize in both; I'll admit my personal bias freely.

It's just that the more you know, the more you can change. Genomic and epigenetic data can inform everyday decisions, sometimes in very surprising ways. Here are a few more examples:

- The Monoamine Oxidase A (MAOA) gene has been observed to predict aggressive behavior in high provocation situations; for this reason, it has earned the nickname "warrior gene."[206]

- The genes TAS1R2 rs3935570 and rs35874116 are associated with a preference for sweet foods.[207]

- Neuroticism has been observed to be 48 percent heritable.[208]

- A lot of evidence exists for alcoholism as genetic, with the specific genes ADH1B and ALDH2 identified as prominent risk factors.[209]

- Even chronotype—when you tend to wake up—is genetically influenced.[210]

- Caffeine metabolism-related genes explain why some people can drink espresso at 9:00 p.m. and sleep soundly while others lie awake for hours as if they'd just blitzed a horror movie marathon. The gene CYP1A2 controls caffeine metabolism; you can be "fast," "medium," or "slow."[211]

- Genetic markers also influence whether your body is better suited to endurance versus explosive sports, whether you thrive as an "early bird" or a "night owl," whether you drink too much, whether you like sweet foods, and so on. Aligning your routines with these predispositions unlocks pure *life*.

You get the idea. Your genes are no verdict, but they are a roadmap. By building your data atop the pillars of sleep, exercise, nutrition, and stress management, you can construct truly resilient health to stand for the rest of your life.

If you would like my clinic's help with genomic and epigenetic data collection and sensemaking, you can schedule a free, no-obligation conversation with us at your convenience at www.velocityhealthclinic. com/bookings.

Extensive Blood Panels

OK, let's pause for a fair question before we proceed. *Could all this just be over-testing?* Now another question. *Just a way to waste time, spread anxiety, and get paid?*

The critiques are real. Extra scans can find things that don't really matter, can trigger unnecessary follow-ups, and cause more stress than overall benefit. Sometimes earlier detection only makes survival look longer without actually changing outcomes. And yes, "incidentalomas"—those random lumps or shadows on a scan—can strike unnecessary terror, spike stress, and worsen other, very real health concerns. So how do we avoid all that?

- Velocity **only** tests when we suspect results will change long-term management. If a number won't alter a decision—nutrition, training, medication, monitoring—we don't need it.

- We **only** pre-commit to decision trees. Before ordering, we tell you, simply, "If X shows up, we do Y. If not, we wait." No drifting into endless follow-ups. No time wasted. No money drained needlessly.

- Velocity **only** uses low-risk tools first. Take DEXA, MRI, and low-dose scans, when appropriate. We reserve the heavier-dose options like CCTA for cases where the benefit outweighs the risk.

- And we **always** pair data with direction. Numbers without context create fear. Numbers with a plan reduce fear because you can watch risk fall over time. That's the Velocity way.

And **all** of that brings us to bloodwork. Unlike speculative scans, blood tests are low-risk, relatively low-cost, and highly actionable. They can uncover silent risks in cholesterol, inflammation, hormones, micronutrients, and more—long before you'd ever know something was wrong. Yes, each takes time, a little pain, and some money, but we believe you are best served by getting most if not all of these. In alphabetical order . . .

The Lab Work Everyone Needs in Midlife

Alongside each entry below is the common listed price of that particular biomarker in the United States. It all adds up to between $500 and $600 once per year. But there are clinics like Velocity Health where you can have a comprehensive look at all of these; plus, you can have a team to help guide you through proper interpretation so you know what they each mean individually, what the numbers mean in concert with each other, and what to do about any causes of concern. Now for the list:

- **Apolipoprotein B**: Assesses cardiovascular health and risk of developing coronary artery disease for $18.

- **CBC with Differential**: Measures blood components for overall health, infections, anemia, and immune issues for $3 - $5.

- **Comprehensive Metabolic Panel (CMP)**: Assesses the health of kidneys, liver, electrolyte and acid/base balance, blood glucose, and blood protein levels for $8.

- **Cortisol**: Assesses stress response and adrenal function for $5 - $7.

- **C-Reactive Protein, HS (CRP, HS)**: Indicator of inflammation and heart disease risk for $10 - $12.

- **Cystatin C**: Assesses kidney function for $14.

- **DHEA-S**: Reflects adrenal gland function for $9.

- **Estradiol (E2)**: Essential for reproductive health for $9 - $12.

- **Ferritin**: Indicates iron storage levels for $12.

- **FSH & LH**: Key hormones in reproductive health for $20.

- **Fructosamine**: Assessment of short-term glycemic control for $12.

- **Hemoglobin A1c**: Long-term indicator of blood sugar control (over 3-month period) for $5.

- **Homocysteine**: Assesses overall health and potential risk for various chronic diseases for $20.

- **IGF-1**: A hormone that manages the effects of growth hormone (GH) in your body for $19 - $22.

- **Insulin, Fasting**: Indicates blood sugar regulation for $16.

- **Iron + Total Iron Binding Capacity**: Assesses Iron status for $10.

- **Lipid Panel**: Assesses cardiovascular health risk for $5.

- **Lipoprotein(a)**: Evaluates lipid metabolism disorders and assesses coronary heart disease for $16.

- **NMR LipoProfile®**: Directly measures the amount of LDL circulating in the body for $50.

- **Progesterone**: Important for menstrual cycle and pregnancy for $4 - $6.

- **PSA, Free and Total**: Prostate-specific Antigen, a protein made by the prostate gland for $10.

- **Prolactin**: Hormone produced by the pituitary gland for $10.

- **Reverse T3**: Evaluates thyroid function, inactive form of T3 for $22.

- **T3, Total**: Evaluates thyroid function, active thyroid hormone for $5.

- **Testosterone, Free & Total w/ SHBG**: Assesses testosterone levels for hormonal balance for $25 - $30.

- **Thyroid Panel**: Evaluates thyroid function for $23.00 - $27.00.

- **Vitamin B12 & Folate**: Essential for nerve function and blood cell formation for $22.00 - $25.00.

- **Vitamin D, 25-OH, Total**: Important for bone health and immune function for $18.00 - $22.00.

Here's what happens when you get the data—the data gets you.

The Numbers Tell the Whole Story

All of the above in this chapter, together with the tests I've shared with you prior throughout the book, will offer you the most comprehensive, accurate state-of-your-health description you've ever seen. You will make sense and make meaning of all the numbers and the complete picture they show, provided you have the expert alongside you (or are one). That's the value of a partner like Velocity—you can order each individually, but what do they mean if you don't have the full and total context? Each new number can tell an entirely different story, but how do you weave all the subplots together to tell the whole story about what's happened to your health and where's it going—and what you can do about it . . . and, possibly, may even have to in order to save your life but no previous doctor caught it?

That's what we do. But our advanced diagnostics at Velocity constantly evolve because so is the field. Here is a break-down of a few such advanced data-gatherers, with prices. These tests all dig deeper into genetic, cellular, and systemic health.

One last remark on these advanced diagnostics. I've heard from some critics that full-body MRIs are not worth it because they ultimately cause more trouble than they're worth via overdiagnosing and overprescribing based on the results.

Velocity has completed hundreds of such scans. Not *once* have we subjected a patient to something unnecessary based on the findings. It was a delicate and detailed discussion about risks, benefits, alternatives, how we would cautiously wait and watch in a structured way.

On the other hand, I've caught four early-stage cancers in young people who would've never been screened (caught at stage 1 and dealt with), diagnosed (for the first time) years-long autoimmune issues, seen early white matter changes that led to altered cognitive plans, and perhaps just as importantly been able to give people piece of mind that nothing huge is underlying (with the caveat we don't see everything, just most of it).

All arguments against advanced therapeutics and testing come down to time and trust more than anything, in my opinion. If you give your patient time to explain everything, and have a relationship built on trust, then you don't go spiraling down these pathways. You are informed and empowered by data to make real actionable change in their lives.

Besides, technology will never stop advancing. It never has and never will. In the next decade, full body MRIs (or some other comprehensive diagnostic) will become so good and so affordable (say, $100 each) that it will just be a yearly thing we all do. The science and technology *will* get there, as it always does. But this is the necessary rubicon we must pass. We have to go through this awkward messy phase before we break down paradigms and create a new standard of care. We will.

Brian and Eric's Stories, Continued

Brian and Eric remind us why measuring what matters is non-negotiable in middle age and beyond. Brian discovered that "fine" masked a cascade of early problems across multiple systems—problems that if left untouched for any number of years more could have landed him in the hospital and left him with fewer years (and less quality of life in those years). By fixing them *now*, Brian not only regained his health but extended his future. Eric, to his own credit, learned that even peak performers can be undermined by invisible risks. The path to best results isn't working harder, it's smarter; sometimes, that means *less* hard. Trite but true.

Both men offer us examples of how advanced diagnostics move us beyond guesswork. Testing deeply, uncovering the hidden weaknesses, and then creating a plan that builds resilience for the long run—this is healthspan optimization. Brian reclaimed vigor for work, family, and the years ahead. Eric unlocked performance he didn't even know he was missing and could access. And both prove the same age-old point: You cannot manage what you do not measure.

As we close this chapter, remember this: Precision testing is not just for elite athletes or affordable only to top executives. It's for anyone who refuses to settle for the four-letter lie of *fine*. Measure what truly matters, and you can give yourself the possibility of a body and a mind that keep pace with your ambitions for decades to come.

CHAPTER 8
Personalized Precision Interventions

Remember Nina from Chapter 1? At 55, she wasn't sick, you might recall, and she was determined to stay that way. Watching her mother struggle with dementia made her resolve to "future-proof" her own brain. We became her partner in that endeavor. So at Velocity, we ran advanced diagnostics—and promptly found that Nina carried one copy of APOE4, a genetic variant linked to higher Alzheimer's risk and had mildly elevated homocysteine, a marker tied to B-vitamin status. With those insights, she got a tailored brain health plan, written around diet, targeted nutrients, and brain-engaging activities, to repeat myself.

Nina's journey, however, didn't stop there. Like many of our patients, she wanted to know what else was possible beyond the Core Four of sleep, nutrition, exercise, and mental resilience. She asked the question you, too, might be asking as you embark on this chapter: *Should I try advanced therapies, things like peptides, rapamycin, hyperbaric oxygen?*

But *"Should I try these?"* is the wrong question. It's too soon, too simplistic. These interventions can be powerful but *only* when introduced at the right time and for the right reasons. Nina's story illustrates the framework we use, the one I've given you over the course of this book. It's basically gone like this: First, we optimize the foundations, which are the Core Four. Without these built up, no futuristic compound or device is likely to save you. Second, we address clear biomarkers of risk from your advanced diagnostics (like Nina's homocysteine). Only with basics nailed and risks under control do we consider advanced therapeutics.

This is the "structured curiosity" that defines Velocity. We aren't a longevity boutique that sells supplements with clickbait promises. We're, in short, the third option. So yes, we sometimes use off-label or experimental tools, but only always with full transparency and a benefit-risk framework (which I'll show you in very short order).

And that's how Nina came to explore therapies like BPC-157 (a peptide studied for tissue repair) and dihexa (an experimental compound targeting brain function). Now, these aren't FDA-approved medications, so they require caution, clear-eyed evaluation, and a specialized client-doctor partnership. But with the Core Four in place and her personalized risks mapped out, Nina could make an informed choice about whether adding advanced interventions fit her health plan. We felt good about exploring what else medical science could offer her.

Let's do the same for you now, but we'll do so in the context of the framework I teased a couple of paragraphs ago. Let's go.

Velocity Health Advanced Therapeutics Decision Framework

This is how we think about personalized precision intervention opportunities. We don't go with instinct, but with a system. This helps us make consistent, defensible, and patient-centered decisions about what to try, when to try it, and how to know if it's working.

And again, foundations come first. No advanced therapy can substitute for the basics. If sleep, nutrition, exercise, and mental resilience aren't addressed—or at least well underway—then the most cutting-edge intervention will not move the needle. In fact, there is a non-zero chance you could get worse if the fundamentals go unaddressed. This is why we hold to transparent safety margins. We prioritize interventions with wide therapeutic windows, clear "stop" rules, and effects we can reverse if needed.

Another thing to keep in mind here. "Precision" is not a marketing word. We believe the right tool has to match the right person at the right time. Just because a compound or therapy is novel or effective in some cases like yours doesn't mean it belongs in your plan. Precision also carries forward from measurement to maintenance. This is non-negotiable. If we can't define what success looks like before we start, we don't start. Every intervention <u>must</u> have outcomes and timelines agreed upon in advance. And if it's not improving the markers we set out to move, we stop.

With these principles in place, let's now walk you through the multi-part decisionmaking framework for how to know what does (or does not) make sense for your unique situation.

Intake → Alignment → Prioritization

When a Velocity patient first explores advanced therapeutics with us, we begin by listening. **Intake** is about uncovering motives. **What are you optimizing for?** Is the goal to train pain-free, to lift your VO_2 max, to extend cognitive stamina, to reverse biological age markers, or simply to look and feel stronger, as common examples?

Next comes **alignment**. Every new therapy comes with uncertainty and potential side effects, so we ask directly what level of risk you are comfortable with. Some are willing to tolerate more unknowns for the chance at a breakthrough; others prefer interventions with a wider safety margin. The answer shapes which options stay on the table.

Finally, **prioritization** finishes the initial stage of precision intervention decisionmaking. With hundreds of possibilities available, what matters most to you *right now*? Together, we define one to three outcomes that are measurable and meaningful, or what we in medicine call "minimum clinically important differences." That could mean, for example, increasing VO_2 max by 10 percent within six months, dropping ApoB cholesterol below 65 mg/dL in four months, or cutting weekly migraine days from six down to two in twelve weeks. Some of these target outcomes will be entirely goal-based to live richly. Others may have an improvement associated with a diagnosis. Still others may relate to symptoms that are suspect. We ask every patient about these before evidence appraisal, which comes next.

Evidence Appraisal (EASI Scoring)

This is where we score each potential therapy (for you) against our EASI to standardize judgment. It looks like this.

Dimension	What We Check	Score (0–3)
E – Evidence Strength	Meta-analyses/RCTs? Effect size consistent? External validity to our patient?	0 none → 3 strong
A – Alignment	Does the mechanism/ outcome align with *this* patient's phenotype, biomarkers, and goals?	0 low → 3 high
S – Safety	Known adverse events, monitoring ease, reversibility, drug–gene (PGx) interactions	0 narrow window → 3 wide
I – Impact	Expected **absolute** benefit on a prioritized outcome (MCID, NNT) and time-to-benefit	0 minimal → 3 major

Interpretation:

- **9–12 → Reasonable to offer now (if patient values fit).**

- **5–8 → Consider within protocol/registry, or after foundations.**

- **0–4 → Not recommended outside study.**

This works. Up next.

Benefit, Harm, Burden Matrix (BHB)

Here, we write a brief one-pager detailing risk-benefit numbers and their natural frequencies. There are several categories which matter. Here you go.

Category	Items
Benefits (absolute)	"Expected VO₂ ↑ ~10% (range 5–15%) in 12–16 weeks" / "ApoB ↓ 30–50 mg/dL by 3 months"
Harms (absolute)	e.g., mouth ulcers in ~10–20% on rapa (dose-dependent); GI upset with metformin ~20%, B12↓ over time
Burden	Time (sessions/week), opportunity cost (what it displaces), financial cost, travel
Uncertainties	Missing human data, long-term unknowns, publication bias, generalizability
Alternatives	Standard options with evidence (and their BHB)
Stop rules	What would make us pause/ stop (biomarker cutoffs, adverse events, no effect by week X)
Monitor	Baseline, cadence, specific labs/ imaging/scores; who reviews and when

By the way, when we talk about all this, the clarity of informed consent is everything. That's why we (try to) avoid vague relative percentages and instead use absolute numbers. For example, "Your risk goes from 10 in 100 down to 6 in 100," rather than "a 40 percent reduction." All this helps you know what, exactly, you would be saying *yes* or *no* to.

We also (as best we can) put results in timeframes so you know when to expect change, such as, "by twelve weeks, we expect to see improvement." Every intervention is tied to minimum clinically important differences (MCIDs) like "a VO_2 max gain of 10 percent or more is significant for you." Thus, all decision-making becomes transparent, personalized, and—as much as possible—safe. (By the way, it's "minimum" because it's the minimum positive change that you *notice*. And we want you to notice important changes!)

Monitoring & Maintenance

Starting is not enough; we need to know if it's working or not. Is it promising, or should we discourage further use? We need to know.

With that goal set in mind already, we'll set a cadence for monitoring, like labs every four to eight weeks, patient-reported outcomes weekly through an app, and device-based metrics daily or weekly. Progress is then evaluated using a decision tree. If the patient meets the pre-specified improvement, they're considered a responder and move into a consolidation phase. If there's no meaningful improvement by the checkpoint, we adjust, escalating dose, switching to a different mechanism, or stopping altogether.

But if there's an adverse event, the rule is simple— pause, evaluate, and follow a structured dechallenge or rechallenge approach before calling it off altogether.

Every therapy must have a stop rule so we know when to quit and don't worsen things. We do not deviate from the rules.

And as an addendum, every check-in should leave an audit trail—brief notes recording the data, interpretation, and action—so the story of progress is always clear and defensible.

OK, let's now look at some examples to see all this in action.

Bringing It All Together

Examples of Precision Medicine Intervention Decisions

Here's how we've objectively assessed if we should test one of these therapeutics—and if we should continue once we do (or stop it).

> **Example: Rapamycin** (Weekly, Low-Dose)
>
> - **Prior/Target:** Healthy 58-year-old optimizer; goal = slow biologic aging, maintain immune vigor.
>
> - **EASI: E2–3 (animal data strong; human aging trials early), A3, S2 (mucositis, lipids; reversible), I1–2 (uncertain absolute benefit; proxy markers).** → *Score 8–10 (Promising/Experimental)*
>
> - **BHB: Benefits (possible epigenetic/immune effects); Harms (mouth ulcers ~10–20%,**

lipids ↑); Burden (labs q8–12 wks);
Unknowns (long-term in healthy humans).

- Stop rules: ulcers refractory; LDL ↑ >30%
  despite management; infections ↑.
- Monitor: lipids, CBC, oral health, infections;
  optional epigenetic age.

Example: Platelet-Rich Plasma (PRP) for Knee
Osteoarthritis (Ultrasound-Guided)

- Prior/Target: 52-year-old lifestyle
  improver; goal = pain ↓, function ↑;
  imaging confirms OA.
- EASI: E3 (meta-analyses > HA/placebo),
  A3, S3 (autologous; low AE), I2–3 (pain/
  function MCIDs common 6–12 mo). →
  Score 11–12 (Standard/Promising)
- BHB: Benefits (pain ↓ in ~60–70% by 6–12
  mo); Harms (injection discomfort); Burden
  (1–3 sessions).
- Stop rules: no functional gain by 12 wks;
  escalate PT or alternative.

Example: Hyperbaric Oxygen Therapy (HBOT)
for Aging/Longevity

- Prior/Target: 65-year-old pre-disease worrier;
  wants cognitive/vascular resilience.
- EASI: E2 (small RCTs showing telomere/
  senescence shifts), A2–3, S3, I2 (functional

proxies). → *Score 9–10 (Promising)*

- **BHB:** Benefits (biologic markers; some cognitive recovery data); Harms (barotrauma risk low); Burden (40–60 sessions).

- **Stop rules:** intolerable barotrauma, no subjective/objective gains by session 20.

Example: Peptide BPC-157 (Injury Healing)

- **Prior/Target:** 49-year-old self-starter with chronic tendinopathy; failed PT/NSAIDs.

- **EASI: E1 (animal/mechanistic; minimal human data), A2, S1–2 (unknown long-term), I1–2.** → *Score 5–7 (Experimental; protocol/registry only)*

- **BHB:** Benefits (theoretical faster tendon healing); Harms (unknown oncologic risks via angiogenesis/FAK); Burden (compounding, monitoring).

- **Stop rules: no improvement by 6–8 weeks; any adverse signal → stop.**

Where are the examples about metformin? NAD+ or stem cells? Hormone replacement therapy? I could write a whole 'nother book on all alternative and advanced therapies. Perhaps I will at some point. Our priority, however, is not to tell you *what* to think of these drugs; it's to teach you *how* to think about them before, during, and/or after trying them. Any of them. All of them.

I <u>cannot</u> recommend any one person try any one of these, and that's why I suggest you meet with a qualified medical professional. I unhumbly again suggest Velocity Health Clinic, now that you know how we'll think through and talk about with you your own goals beyond the Core Four. Again, the link is www. velocityhealthclinic.com/bookings.

Now, you might already be optimized, needing no three- to six-month waiting period to get your sleep etc. in order. That's the case for a few Velocity patients. One of them, a retired Major League Soccer player now in his sixties, came to us with a clear mission—he wants to live to 110 and beyond. His training is impeccable, his sleep is dialed in, his relationships are strong. Because his foundation is so solid, he's eager to explore almost every frontier therapy available—rapamycin, as well as dasatinib plus quercetin (a protocol being studied by Mayo Clinic researchers that reduces neuroinflammation and lower Alzheimer's risk, though as of this writing, it is still pre-clinical), and more.[212]

Within a month of working with us, we were already having thoughtful conversations about these compounds. He's now layering on additional modalities like peptides and hyperbaric oxygen, while we track his labs closely and apply strict stop-rules if anything looks unsafe. He knows some of this carries unknowns—we're transparent about what science supports, what's emerging, and what's speculative—but he accepts the risks in exchange for the potential upside.

In many ways, he's the closest we've seen to a Bryan Johnson type—a super-collector of data who wants to test, measure, and optimize everything. Johnson, in case you don't know, is "the world's most measured man" and tracks dozens of biomarkers to strengthen his longevity, treating his health not as luck but as a trackable system that can be improved upon.[213] Per a 2023 *Time* magazine article, Bryan Johnson's explicit goal is bigger than our ex-soccer player's; Johnson wants to live forever:

> "Most people assume death is inevitable. We're just basically trying to prolong the time we have before we die," he says. Until now, he adds, "I don't think there's been any time in history where Homo sapiens could say with a straight face that death may not be inevitable."[214]

I was part of an intimate discussion that Bryan Johnson had with a group of physician investors not long before authoring this book. I published my thoughts shortly afterwards; here are some excerpts:

> An interesting thought experiment he posed to many leading up to his Don't Die movement: if we were in 2050, and human life was profoundly blissful, what would we say, looking back, were some of the most important and foundational cultural movements that fundamentally shifted the course of humanity? What could we then each do right now that would move that vision forward? After dozens of dinners w [sic] dozens of folks hearing them talk about this, he landed on Don't Die, which he sees as the

new "operating system" for humanity. The explosion of AI and scientific progress will come sooner and more powerfully than we understand. Harnessing this velocity into positive human health is the idea he wants to be remembered for - a worthy and audacious goal.

. . . One thing that must happen if our society truly embraces Don't Die is a Zeitgeist of cultural and social change. We need to hold up the pinnacle of health as just as important pillars vs wealth, power, status, influence, etc. We need all of our friends and families obsessed with health and striving every day to make it better. The second and third order effect of that will be profound, but is foundational to embracing this idea.

One interesting offshoot from this part of discussion: Bryan understands that data is cloudy and we don't study the things that matter most. Part of the Don't Die movement is also a foundation that's been set up to conduct large scale studies on lifestyle and other interventions that don't typically get funded in our current paradigm.

. . . Ultimately, he concedes that NONE of us have any idea how the future will play out. Maybe a year from now, 10 years from now, 50 years from now, we'll each want to die. But as he says, the goal is:

"Don't die right now"

Which resonates with me. We each deserve to understand our bodies and health precisely and to live up to the full potential of our existence. Performing as the very best version of ourself [sic] RIGHT NOW is really the goal.

We will need many along this journey to tell the story in their own way. I'm glad there are so many m nodes of activity in this space and continue to welcome the robust dialogue.

Even if "don't die" doesn't resonate with you - LIVE NOW is something I think many of us can get behind.[215]

Advanced and experimental therapies are interesting, but let's not make them a detracting distraction. I =can't stress this enough . . . whether it's with Velocity or another clinic, please, **please** do not attempt any of these therapeutics, drugs, or advanced treatments until you've got the basics in order. Just take testosterone replacement therapy (TRT) as an example of why.

The most common scenario I see is men eager to jump straight to TRT even though they're still fifty to a hundred pounds overweight, sleeping poorly, eating terribly, not exercising, and often stuck in toxic relationships. In that state, more testosterone won't fix the problem—it can actually make things worse. That's because excess fat tissue contains an enzyme called aromatase, which converts testosterone into estrogen.

Instead of feeling better, these men end up with serious estrogen-related side effects.

That's why we set baseline requirements. Before we even discuss advanced therapeutics, patients need to show they're consistently working on those all-important Core Four. Do I need to go through them again? Probably not. But let's do it anyway. They are . . .

Sleep.

Nutrition.

Training.

Mental resilience.

In any particular order, in any order. Because for most, the first three to six months are spent gathering data, addressing fundamentals, and building healthier patterns in *all* of them, and all at once as best we are able. Only after doing so can we say the foundation is in place can we explore whether adding something like TRT—or any other advanced therapy—makes sense for the new you that you want to build.

Mindset matters here, too, particularly in the case of TRT. If someone's relationships are strained or their mental state is unstable, pushing their hormones artificially can amplify the worst parts of their behavior. That's why we encourage open conversations with partners, careful reflection on mindset, and active work on relationships before jumping in. Otherwise, advanced therapeutics become more of a liability than a solution.

All that to say, when you are truly ready, you'll know it. Like Nina.

Nina's Story, Continued

For Nina, her focus became lowering inflammation, especially the subtle neurological inflammation that can quietly erode brain health over time (remember the dementia worries). Now, her foundation was already strong; she slept well, ate a Mediterranean-style diet, and exercised consistently. That meant she had **earned the right** to layer in more advanced therapeutics.

Rather than trying everything for the sake of novelty, we matched therapies to her specific risks—APOE4 status, elevated homocysteine, and family history of dementia. Together, we built a precision brain health plan that included BPC-157 and dihexa, but also high-dose omega-3s. Each intervention targeted a different "lever" so to speak, like lowering systemic inflammation, protecting neurons, and enhancing focus and cognitive stamina.

The result was not only sharper energy and more focus day to day but also a longer-term hedge against the very disease that turned Nina onto health and fitness priorities in the place. Nina worked our system, and now it's working for her.

CHAPTER 9
Sustain and Elevate with Concierge Support

By now, you've learned all the essentials—how to understand your body, how to think through diagnostics, and how to explore advanced therapeutics. The next step is bigger than any one test or treatment. It's about the **structure** of your care.

Here's what I mean by that. Navigating the American healthcare system on your own is like trying to win a championship without a coach, without a playbook, without a team. The system is fragmented, confusing, and often hostile to people who simply want to stay healthy. That's why concierge precision medicine matters. We pull together the right people and the right processes so you don't waste energy, time, and money trying to connect dots on your own.

Outside the concierge experience, and back in the usual system, primary care is reduced to fifteen-minute visits and reactive triage. Specialists work in silos, each looking at their one organ system, leaving you waiting months for conflicting advice. The wellness market is trend-driven, often unregulated, and overwhelming. Diagnostics are episodic—a lab slip here, a PDF there—with no one really synthesizing the story. Digital health apps track everything and, often, integrate nothing.

The result is that otherwise intelligent, motivated adults still feel lost. The system is a disassembly line. No quarterback, no continuous optimization, no one owning the outcome. The way I see it, there are **seven consistent fail points** where the system breaks down; these are the gaps of modern healthcare:

- **Information Gap**: The data exists; insights don't.

- **Coordination Gap**: No one integrates across labs, specialists, and lifestyle.

- **Continuity Gap**: Every new provider resets your health story to zero.

- **Accountability Gap**: There are no shared metrics or follow-through.

- **Context Gap**: Advice rarely accounts for your goals, season of life, or environment.

- **Capacity Gap**: High performers don't have time to project-manage their own care.

- **Community Gap**: Without peers on the same journey, habits don't stick.

A true concierge ecosystem must be built to close every one of these gaps. We do that at Velocity with what we call, aptly, your "T.E.A.M.," which stands for:

- **Translator** – turns complex diagnostics into plain, actionable steps.

- **Engineer** – designs the intervention stack, from nutrition to peptides to training.

- **Accountability Partner** – ensures execution, feedback, and iteration.

- **Monitor** – continuously tracks both objective data and subjective signals.

(Internally, at Velocity, the Translator is the concierge staff, the Engineer is the physician, the Accountability Partner is your health coach, and the Monitor is data-driven disciplinary care. Your T.E.A.M.)

Of course, every member reports to one person: **you**, the patient CEO. And yet each remains accountable to the others. The differentiator is having a single unified operating picture across medical, performance, and purpose. And over time, you can expect your T.E.A.M. to provide the **Five Dimensions of Sustained Optimization**; the seven gaps generally map onto these five, as in, these five dimensions collectively close those seven gaps:

1. **Continuity** — care never resets.
2. **Proactivity** — act before failure.
3. **Integration** — one story, not many notes.
4. **Visibility**— all metrics and scorecards.
5. **Belonging** — reinforcement through tribe and coaching.

Now, these all come off as abstract. I'll explain to you their real, tangible value on your health journey in this way—as the **emotional economics of support**.

You see, without a team, inputs conflict, confidence wavers, momentum stalls, and decision fatigue sets in. With concierge support, there's one narrative, twenty-four-seven access, compounding progress, and freedom from the cognitive load of managing everything yourself. Often, the psychological payoffs—security, focus, agency—can be even greater than the biological one. You have medical practitioners who are watching out for and over you weekly, even daily, as opposed to a few minutes from a distracted, overworked general practitioner once a year at an annual physical (if that).

In my view, this is obviously superior to traditional healthcare. And for most, it's even affordable. Velocity Health offers different membership levels—from essentials, to full diagnostic reviews, to invite-only full-team optimization. But whether you join us or build your own system, the principle is the same: You likely cannot reach peak performance alone. I can't. No one can.

This is the way to sustain and increase your progress.

Now let's learn the advantage the concierge system gives you.

The Concierge Advantage

In the current US health care system, you are on your own. And I don't just mean in terms of payment. You may have insurance, and you may have a primary care physician. This primary care doctor is probably skilled and has taken great care of you.

But the primary care physician can only do so much.

Depending on your medical condition, you'll need a specialist. You'll get a referral, and you'll visit. The care will be pretty good there, too; the specialists know how to treat their patients.

But two months later, when your old health problem is well behind you, a new one pops up. You'll have to see *another* specialist, or maybe even the same one as before. But not only will you need another referral, you're at the mercy of that specialist's schedule. It's better to resolve a health problem sooner rather than later, but both your general practitioner and your specialists have other patients to see, patients that made appointments of their own. So then you search on your own for specialists, but how do you know which ones are worth your time or your money, and will they even take your insurance?

And let's say you do get through to these specialists. You can tell them what other doctors said, show them lab results, and all sorts of things. But will they be able to connect the dots? There's no guarantee of that. And this whole thing is a process that can take *years.*

Concierge medicine changes all that. With a concierge model of care, you get everything under one roof, for the price of a membership; in other words, you're subscribing to your health care. You get health care practitioners with experience in different aspects of health, and they work together to give you a complete picture of your status.

Too often, people waste years of their lives and thousands of dollars trying to knock out one symptom at a time, and in that time, other symptoms arise. By contrast, the concierge approach treats the body as the interconnected system that it is, and recognizes that trouble in one area often means trouble somewhere you would think is unrelated. And because everyone is in one place, you can handle a health problem right when it's detected; no more bouncing from specialist to specialist, none of whom has the complete picture. You save time, which may save your life as well.

The Mechanics of Concierge Medicine

Concierge medicine relies on an interdisciplinary team of physicians who are not only familiar with different aspects of the body, but how they all come together. Instead of just picking one component and saying that "this is everything," they check everything upstream and downstream of that. Sluggishness may not merely be a blood sugar problem, but possibly a cancer problem. Trouble with your eyes may be due to poor nutrition. Poor sexual performance may be due to physical activity levels, not just hormonal imbalances. You may even find an issue where you never thought to look. This is the advantage of an interdisciplinary team.

The best part is that the specialists aren't narrowly focused on their area of expertise. It's not a case where you go to the expert in one thing, then that expert passes a note along to the other one and you go there, and so on. Instead, there are integrated sub-specialists who know not only their area of expertise, but have some knowledge of related areas, too.

For example, let's say you're seeing a cardiologist due

to your high blood pressure. This cardiologist will not only be knowledgeable about cardio but about various diets like the ketogenic diet or the Mediterranean diet and their effect on the body. They'd know how to use various nutrition strategies to help you solve your health problem.

So you may not even need the nearby specialists; the one you're working with will be enough, and this saves you precious time. This is what separates the concierge approach from the usual practice. No chasing referrals. No going from specialist to specialist hoping the new one would know something. No worries about whether or not the specialists would take your insurance. Just all the care you need, all in one place.

Thus the best kind of care, preventative care, comes easy. As the saying goes, an ounce of prevention is worth a pound of cure, and the best time to catch a medical problem is before it becomes a crisis. Without concierge care, you have to navigate innumerable schedules while your health, and thus your life, hangs in the balance.

But with all of this, the question remains: How will insurance handle it? This is where we get to the best part: You don't need to worry about that. The concierge model sidesteps insurance.

Paying for Your Health

Consider how health care is paid for now. Most people who have health insurance get it through their employer. The practitioner you go to has to be within the network of your insurer. You need to know what procedures are covered so that you're not paying through the nose for something vital. It is well-known that medical debt creates an untold financial strain on the American people. Despite 90 percent of Americans having some form of health insurance, 6 percent of adults owe over $1,000 in medical debt.[216] Over half of US adults say they would be unable to pay a sudden $500 medical bill without borrowing money.[217] According to the Bureau of Labor Statistics, ""[t]he median annual premium for civilian workers was $1,560.00 for single coverage medical care benefits and $6,099.12 for family coverage", assuming an employer-sponsored plan.[218] The real, full cost is $9,325 for single coverage and $26,993 for family coverage.[219] Add that on top of having to chase down specialists one at a time, and things get very pricey, very fast.

But when you think about it, you realize that this model is at odds with how we typically think of insurance. "Insurance" is supposed to be something you pay into so that you can get that money back when catastrophe strikes. You get auto insurance in case your car is damaged. You get homeowner's insurance in case your house burns down or some other disaster befalls your home.

But health insurance is different, because taking care of your body is not some rare occurrence, but something you're supposed to do every day. The purpose of your coverage is not to just pay for your care when you experience a sudden threat to your health, such as a grievous wound or a cancer diagnosis. It is for day-to-day checkups and chronic conditions as well.

In other words, not insurance at all, more like a

subscription. So the concierge system just cuts out the insurance middleman and has you pay directly. Instead of paying some gigantic insurance company, you pay the concierge service directly, each month, for your everyday health care needs. From here, you can then switch to a health care plan that covers catastrophic health events, thus acting like other types of insurance. From here, you get real peace of mind, and a health care solution that won't destroy you financially.

And it leads to the question we'll take up next: *If concierge care can transform one person's life, what would it look like if we redesigned the entire American healthcare system around its underlying practices and principles?*

Let's find out.

CHAPTER 10
Vision for a New American Healthcare

In Chapter 9, I talked about the gaps in the healthcare system and the available stopgaps outside, alongside, or otherwise in parallel to the system. Velocity, among other personalized precision medicine clinics, offers such paths. But let's humor ourselves for a moment as we wonder, *What would actual positive systemic reform look like? How would we design the American healthcare system from the ground up if all of these principles were baked in from day one?*

Consider the thought experiment. Let's hit it where it hurts—and follow the money first.

Incentives All the Way Down

The health industry is broken because health insurance is broken. That said, do we really want a single payer system where the government owns everything? No, I don't think so. Consider CMS, the umbrella over Medicare and Medicaid and their innumerable inefficiencies and wastes. Perhaps Nordic countries work when they pull off socialized medicine, but we are not them. Those countries have the equivalent population of one B-tier U.S. city's metropolitan area.

Meanwhile, here in the States, we've erected a bureaucratic hurdle that only the biggest publicly traded health insurers can meet—a legalized oligopoly—and we pour premiums into for-profit companies. The Affordable Care Act has siphoned *$9 trillion* out of the economy to large insurers.[220] This is not ideal, according to this citizen.

One of the most frustrating aspects downstream of all this corruption is, of course, pricing. American healthcare is the only industry in the world where you have no idea what the price of any service will be before you get it. You can't shop, can't counter, can't argue after the fact; third parties set it all. This isn't unique to healthcare; it is unique to American healthcare because the two people actually in the interaction—the physician and the patient—are divorced from the economic relationship:

- The patient has an employer; their health care depends on employment.

- The employer pays a health insurer.

- The insurer pays a health system.

- The health system pays a salary to an employed doc.

As of January 2024, 77.6 percent of US physicians are employed by a big health system or corporate entity.[221]

Of those roughly 1 million licensed US physicians, 90,000 of them are affiliated with the huge provider UnitedHealth through its arm Optum, with 10,000 of those 90,000 directly employed by them.[222, 223] That's almost 10 percent! So the incentives are all messed up. Doctors are incentivized to treat patients like widgets, to see more volume because that's how their overlords compensate them. Do more stuff, get paid more.

You should probably know that we in America have a committee in Congress set by the American Medical Association, which is a corrupt organization, called the RUC (the Relative Value Scale Update Committee). They recommend the prices for how much a doctor gets paid for every single different procedure, though the Centers for Medicare and Medicaid Services (CMS) make the final decision.[224] There are tens of thousands of CPT codes, and every year a shadowy group gets in a room and decides how much you're going to pay a doctor to do a cardiac cath versus have a conversation about changing your diet. They set those rates, it permeates the system, and dictates how everyone gets paid. Commercial insurers often go higher.[225] And that's not to mention mass healthcare provider consolidation driving up prices, as most monopolies and oligopolies tend to do. The excuse is "increased administrative costs," according to the professionals who work in the non-clinical departments of these large organizations. In reality, it's about profit, pure and simple. And that's when you see major networks slapping their name and logo on all the various small providers in town that you used to know by another name. They sold; some, you could say, sold out.

With that context, you can see how the cost of care has become separate from the quality of care in this country—and no amount of tinkering is going to change us. We've tried incremental change for fifty years, and yet 70 percent of us are overweight or obese and 60 percent have diabetes. The system is broken and needs replacement. Here's what we might consider.

Bottom-Up System Correction

We need a total overhaul. Here are three ideas for exactly that:

1. Individualized, "n=1" prevention-first care tailored to each person's body and life.
2. Cash-pay environment for procedures and specialists to unleash real competition.
3. Catastrophic coverage with no confusing networks—true insurance for the bad stuff.

Let's start with *n=1*, which simply means the number is one. One patient. One priority.

In modernity, our lives are infinitely complex—culture, preferences, lifestyle, support, family history, genetics, environmental exposures, labs. When a clinician glances at a basic panel and says "you're fine," we all know that's not comprehensive. The *n=1* care correction means each person is unique and deserves tailored healthcare. It requires time, deep intake, and interdisciplinary teams (doctors, dietitians, strength and conditioning coaches, mental health professionals, etc.) to build long-term plans. Early data suggest *n=1* increases patient satisfaction and improves community-level outcomes in obesity and diabetes through early screening, counseling, and prevention emphasis.

It also means addressing SDOH (which stands for food security, physical exercise, psychosocial well-being). A program called **Healthy People 2030** is a start, with a goal to "[set] data-driven national objectives to improve health and well-being over the next decade" by measuring not only traditional health indicators, but the social determinants of health as well.[226] If we prioritize holistic well-being over symptom-chasing, we can avert disease before it arises.

Next up is **cash pay**. Look, we don't have real competition in healthcare. Prices are hidden until after the fact—when patients are most vulnerable. Ask how much a basic test costs and most working in the system will say, "It depends," or, "I can't answer that." Every price is obfuscated behind insurer contracts you'll never see. We've allowed too many middlemen into the sacred patient-clinician relationship; at every step, dollars are extracted without value added.

So let's just delete the middle layers. And let physicians and patients engage in direct commerce, competing on quality, cost, and experience.

Cash pay streamlines payment, reduces admin waste, and forces price transparency. Until then, always ask the cash price before you use insurance.

We've got to do something about those premiums. **Catastrophic coverage** is the only thing affordable to most American families now, reasonably speaking, and that's OK. Consider a metaphor I introduced earlier—car insurance. Do you use car insurance for an oil change? For a carburetor? No. You buy maintenance out of pocket and reserve insurance for accidents. Health should be the same. Use insurance only for the truly catastrophic—new cancer, major trauma, surgeries, hospitalizations. By law, hospitals have to treat acute conditions regardless of patient ability to pay (good), but the unpaid bills crush families (bad).

So, let's insure claims over $10,000. That safety net prevents bankruptcy while giving people control over day-to-day care. It offers peace of mind, more choice, more purchasing power, and more money to invest in wellness. It also saves billions, possibly trillions, by stripping out prior-auth purgatory and surprise bills. Insurers shouldn't decide appropriate care—you and your doctor should. Insurers should only prevent financial ruin when catastrophe strikes.

And we technically don't necessarily need insurance companies to handle catastrophic coverage. Health cost crowdsharing nonprofits, including religious ministries, have stepped up to offer families welcome alternatives. These are here to stay. Good.

So all in all, there are steps each of us can take to slowly change our healthcare system, one decision at a time. But systematically speaking, total industry transformation is a tall order. It's possible, but it won't be easy. We must build new organizations and networks. We must get highly personalized *n=1* care to every person in ways that make sense. We must retool specialty and procedural platforms so cash-pay and transparency reign. And we must go head-to-head with the health gangsters—the big insurers and incumbents who don't want a brighter future.

Until then, many of us are committed to creating an alternative system that patients and providers can safely eject into—to escape the machine and find true healthcare that serves their needs.

And due to **artificial intelligence**, I don't believe we'll have a choice. Until the highest-tech future fully arrives, we have a window—and a responsibility— to get ready. Track the markers that actually predict outcomes. Make decisions grounded in evidence, guided by judgment, and supported by real relationships. You may not be able to change the system, but you can change yourself. If you'd like to start your *n=1* plan, measure what matters, and protect your ultimate asset, please consider visiting www.velocityhealthclinic.com/ bookings today.

The Ultimate Asset

Afterword by Joshua Lisec

New York Times Bestselling Author & Dr. Deep's Writing
Partner

• • • •

Allow me to introduce myself. I'm Dr. Deep's writing
partner for *The Ultimate Asset*; I am more than this,
however. I'm a contributor to the entire field of health
and wellness book publishing. You've likely read many
prior works of mine. I've been writing for physicians
since 2011, ghostwritten more than 110 nonfiction
books for doctors, researchers, clinicians, dieticians,
nutritionists, registered nurses, personal trainers, fitness
coaches, alternative health practitioners, and allopaths
and naturopaths alike.

Now, that's not a brag so much as a disclosure. I'm
not a doctor. I'm not a dietitian. I'm not your clinician.
I am the guy they call when they finally say, "I can't
not say this out loud anymore. I need the book that tells
the whole truth."

From my vantage point at the intersection of
medicine, publishing, and science communication for
the general public, I've watched something profound
change over the last decade and a half. The marketing
language around health has changed, yes—but so have
the questions patients ask, and the kind of doctor who's
brave enough to answer them honestly.

The system doesn't cut it anymore. For most people,

the pattern goes like this:

"I have a problem."

You notice symptoms. Aches. Fatigue. Brain fog. Weight gain that doesn't respond to what always worked before. Sleep that won't cooperate. Mood swings that don't feel like "you."

You bring these symptoms to your doctor. Maybe you get a little counseling on "root cause"—stress, age, genetics, lifestyle. If you get labs at all, they're usually shallow versions of what's actually possible. You're told you're "fine." Maybe borderline. Maybe "keep an eye on this." But basically, fine. And yet you don't feel fine, as Dr. Deep recounts what Velocity Health patients share when they arrive at his digital doorstop.

Over the years, the various doctors and healthcare professionals I've worked with as their ghostwriter or editor all wanted to write some version of the same book. At its core, each one was really saying:

"This is all the stuff I want to be able to tell my patients or clients, but there just isn't time inside the system."

Many of them went into private practice so they could create that time for their people, while others went big and mainstream with their book to reach the patient they would never meet in person. The motivated forty-something. The exhausted fifty-something. The sixty-something who refuses to accept that "slowing down" and "falling apart" are synonyms.

Still others had a mission to undo what they'd done. I co-authored the 2024 *New York Times* bestseller *Lies I Taught in Medical School* with Robert Lufkin, MD to do just that. That book is a confession and a reckoning.

Dr. Lufkin "lied" about many common medical problems, such as diabetes:

> Sugar is harmless, other than causing weight gain and tooth decay.[227]

. . . and cancer:

> Most cancer is caused by accumulated DNA damage.[228]

. . . and even mental health:

> Metabolism has little effect on mental health.[229]

And finally, he did all the right things in his youth—follow the food pyramid, eat low fat and high carbs, replace saturated fat with seed oils, and even eat only the white of the egg. He followed all the "correct" medical advice for much of his life . . . until he got slammed with high blood pressure, gout arthritis, and prediabetes.[230] In other words, he fell victim to his own "lies" or rather, those myths of the medical establishment. It's a physician saying, *I followed the rules, and the rules were wrong. Here's how I know, and here's what to do instead.*

When you help write that kind of book, you don't walk away the same as you went in. You can't spend hundreds of hours inside the mind of a doctor who has seen the system from the inside, who has watched people get sicker despite "doing everything right," and not begin to question your own assumptions about health, disease, and aging.

That's where my "professional life" as a ghostwriter and my personal life as a human with a body collided.

10 Years a Vegan (And How I Became My Own Guinea Pig)

My own health view has been through a decade-long trial by fire. Ten years a vegan, to low-carb omnivore. Now, when I say "ten years a vegan," I don't mean the half-hearted version with mostly soymilk but the occasional whey protein shake and maybe some bone broth with my beans. I mean the serious, committed, "I'm doing this for the animals and for the planet" version. Imagine the most campy plant-based propaganda, and I publicly pushed it. I bought the promise that if you just ate plants—only plants, the right plants—you could hack your way into a best-case scenario for your body.

About five years in, I started to see the signs . . . I was wrong. Oh, so wrong. Low HDL. High LDL. High triglycerides. Fasting blood glucose level indicating elevated risk of insulin resistance, prediabetes, and type-2 diabetes, and more. For someone who was doing "everything right," my body seemed to be quietly preparing a rebellion.

I received counsel from my client (I was his writing partner on *Stay Off My Operating Table*) and now friend and co-author Philip Ovadia, MD (our jointly authored work is the spinoff to that first book, entitled *Stay Off My Kitchen Table*) to focus on the low-carb diet. He warned me that I was unable to create a best-case health scenario out of veganism.

He suggested high protein, additional supplements.

I tried those. Awful. Bloating. Zero improvement in the metrics that actually matter. And as years went on, something else happened that hit closer to home than any lab marker.

I began working out three times a week, strength training with kettlebells. I did the work. I showed up. I lifted. I recovered. I did the progressive overload thing you're supposed to do. I could not put on muscle. Then I developed an autoimmune thyroid issue.

Oh, no . . .

That's the cleaned-up version of what I actually said. I spoke with Dr. Ovadia again, my own personal healthcare professionals within the mainstream system, a certified nutritionist, and a handful of alternative health practitioners—and every single one told me it was time to go. End veganism.

By then, I'd developed brain fog, memory loss, chronic fatigue, and worse. This wasn't about abs or aesthetic anything. This was about whether my brain would still be there for my kids in twenty years. Whether my energy would still be there for my work, my family, my responsibilities. All of it. All of everything.

Within approximately six weeks of a low-carb diet, **all** of that was gone. Eggs and whey with collagen powder full-fat dairy smoothie. Cheese and sliced deli meat with either sprouted grain bread or two lettuce leaves as the un-buns. Ground beef or turkey with peppers or onions mixed in. Very simple. Trying different spices and herbs now. Slowly but surely seeing numbers improve.

That's the glamorous reality of healthspan. Small, unsexy, consistent decisions that you repeat not because

they're on a motivational poster but because the data—
and your lived experience—tell you they work. It also
tells you strict plant-based diets probably don't. Here are
the top ten risks associated with vegan diets:

1. Vitamin B12 Deficiency

Vegans don't get enough Vitamin B12. The main
source of this vitamin is meat, poultry, and eggs—all
non-vegan food sources.[231] The lack of this vitamin is
linked to various health problems such as numbness
of feet, difficulty walking, and even memory loss and
dementia. Those who choose a vegan diet require outside
supplementation:

> Elevated rates of vitamin B12 deficiency,
> up to 80%, are observed in populations
> in Hong Kong and India, particularly
> among people following a vegan diet with
> limited inclusion of fortified foods or
> supplementation. As an exclusive animal-
> derived nutrient, vitamin B12 is absent in
> vegan diets, necessitating supplementation
> or fortified plant-based alternatives such as
> plant milk, cereals, and nutritional yeast.
> Although the established daily recommended
> dietary allowance for adults in the United
> States is 2.4 microgrammes of vitamin B12,
> research suggests that due to variations in
> the absorption and utilization of vitamin B12
> from plant sources, vegans might require

higher doses of this vitamin. Therefore, regular monitoring of vitamin B12 levels and adaptive supplementation strategies become imperative to maintain optimal health.[232]

2. Vitamin D Deficiency

While Vitamin D is produced by the skin when sunlight hits it, this natural method doesn't work as well during winter or at higher latitudes. By avoiding animal-based foods, vegans are unable to supplement their Vitamin D. Too little of this vitamin can cause low bone density and premature bone aging.[233]

3. Calcium Deficiency

Most vegans do not get enough calcium, with their intake being below the recommendation of 750 mg per day. Extremely low levels of calcium are linked with an increased likelihood of bone fractures.[234]

4. Increased Anemia Risk

Due to inadequacies in how much vitamin B12, iron, calcium, vitamin D, Iodine, zinc, and omega-3 fatty acids vegans get, the risk of anemia is greater.[235]

5. Zinc Deficiency

Vegan diets do not have enough zinc.[236] This can cause

hair loss, loss of appetite, and low sperm count, among other conditions.[237]

6. Lower Bone Mineral Density

Vegans and vegetarians have lower bone mineral density in the femoral neck and lumbar spine areas, as well as a greater risk of bone fractures (likely from this reduced bone density.)[238]

7. Depression Risk

Vegans are at a moderately increased risk for depression.[239]

8. Protein Deficiency

As you might expect, vegans don't get enough protein.[240] And that lack of protein can cause mood swings, hair, nail, and skin problems, and weakness and fatigue.[241]

9. Iodine Deficiency

Vegans don't get enough iodine either.[242] Iodine deficiency leads to pregnancy complications as well as a slower metabolism due to hypothyroidism, which leads to fatigue and weight gain.[243]

10. Stunted Growth in Children

For children on vegan diets, there is a risk of their growth being hampered, especially in light of the bone density problems that vegan diets can cause.[244]

I can't imagine how worse off I would be long term had I adopted the vegan diet during adolescence. Even as an adult, I was a guinea pig, but I was a wild guinea pig, not domesticated within the system. So I took my health into my own hands and sought out various practitioners and pieced together what would work and whom I could trust. No more veganism for Joshua!

And that's where the story of this book and the story of my health intersect. You see, for most people, this is impossible. Most people don't have a dozen physicians, nutritionists, and specialists in their contact list. Most people don't have access to the latest research through their ghostwriting projects. Most people don't have the time, energy, or bandwidth to cross-compare one clinician's theory against another's, then track the lab results and see what actually changed in their body.

They shouldn't have to. Clinics like Velocity Health bring that all in-house.

What the Future of Healthcare Actually Looks Like

Dr. Deep is the future of healthcare. What he's building at Velocity is more than a nice clinic in a nicer part of town, only done online. Velocity is a cutting-edge prototype for what medicine looks like when you stop assuming people are interchangeable and start treating their biology as a high-value asset.

Most people's experience of healthcare feels like standing outside a locked door, hoping someone on the other side has time for them. With Velocity, it feels like being invited behind the scenes. You're not getting generic advice; you're getting the same level of strategic thinking a physician uses on his own body and family, but applied to your life.

In plain terms . . . you get access to physician-grade strategies and insights designed to extend your healthspan, not just your lifespan. This is simply the practical reality of how the care is structured.

Velocity is a true concierge model for people who demand more from their healthcare. It's powered by two things most patients never get at the same time, (1) deep diagnostics and (2) deep thinking. On one side, you have tools that actually see you—tests that measure your heart, your metabolism, your inflammation, your body composition, your genetics. On the other side, you have an expert physician team that knows how to interpret all of that and turn it into a plan you can live with.

Healthcare, in this world, isn't one-size-fits-all. It's built around the idea that your story, your stressors, your genetics, and your goals make you a category of one.

That's why the diagnostic process looks nothing like the fifteen-minute annual physical you're used to. It might include:

- Advanced blood biomarker panels that go far beyond the usual "cholesterol and sugar" snapshot.

- Genetic and epigenetic analysis to understand your inherited risks and how your lifestyle is turning them on—or off.

- Full body and organ-specific imaging when appropriate—up to and including full-body MRI and advanced heart screens.

- VO$_2$ max testing to gauge how well your cardiovascular system actually performs under stress.

- DEXA scans to quantify muscle, fat distribution, and bone health across your frame.

- Emerging tools like liquid biopsies that hint at trouble long before traditional screening would catch it.

Now, the point is not to drown you in data. The point is to put a spotlight on the handful of signals that actually predict whether your next ten to twenty years will be lived in strength or in slow-motion crisis.

Here's where it gets interesting. Secure AI is part of the ecosystem too, and when done right, it's less "robot doctor" and more "second opinion that never sleeps."

By the way, I ran select parts of my own medical history past AI, and it suggested veganism as the cause if not primary contributor to my thyroid issues—which my human medical workers then confirmed as a likely correlation. That doesn't mean the machine replaces the clinician. It means a smart system can help catch patterns faster, flag outliers sooner, and get the right questions in front of the right expert.

Velocity takes that hybrid approach seriously. Physician and AI-powered insights, working together, see you clearly so you can act early.

But diagnostics are just the front door. From there, the work becomes designing a personal health strategy around your actual biology. That might mean a phased plan that addresses your most urgent risks first—cardiometabolic health, for example—while also mapping out how to improve your sleep, your muscle mass, your mental resilience, your nutrition, and your environment over the next year.

Critically, it doesn't stop after one heroic push. Your health is always evolving; your plan has to evolve with it. Velocity's model assumes that your life will change—your job, your stress, your family responsibilities, your goals. Labs will shift. Hormones will shift. Seasons will change. Instead of treating those shifts as failures, the clinic treats them as expected waypoints.

That's what "ongoing optimization" actually means here:

- Regular check-ins that look at your data, your symptoms, and your lived experience together.

- Adaptive plans that are adjusted when your numbers, your goals, or your reality on the ground change.

- A concierge-level relationship where you're not an anonymous chart, but a known human with a trajectory everyone is paying attention to.

All of this stands in direct contrast to the current system. The way most of us experience healthcare today—life without a Velocity-style model—looks like this:

- **Reactive by default**: Up to 80 percent of chronic disease is preventable, yet the machinery of healthcare spins up only after you're already in trouble. The priority is managing illness, not preventing it.

- **Fragmented care**: One specialist looks at your heart. Another looks at your hormones. Another glances at your labs. They rarely speak to each other, and almost no one is tasked with putting the pieces together into a coherent story about you.

- **No personalization**: You're treated like a demographic, not like a person. Age, sex, and one or two risk factors stand in for your actual physiology and history.

- **Insurance-first incentives**: Reimbursement rules reward quick visits and high-code interventions, not the slow, daily work of helping someone stay out of the hospital for the next twenty years.

Now, I don't believe anyone intentionally designed the system to sabotage your healthspan. But as it currently exists, it's not designed to maximize that healthspan.

Velocity's answer is to flip those assumptions. Life with a clinic like this looks like:

- **Integrated diagnostics**: Your data isn't scattered; it's curated. Complex test results are simplified into clear, actionable insights that tell you exactly where you stand and what matters most right now.

- **Individualized strategies**: Your plan isn't pulled from a template. It's built from your numbers, your narrative, and your ambitions. Expertise, secure AI, and your own feedback loop combine to fine-tune your path.

- **Adaptive, responsive care**: Your team doesn't just hand you a binder and wish you luck. They monitor your progress and adjust your protocol when life inevitably throws you curveballs.

- **Direct-pay freedom**: By stepping outside traditional insurance constraints, they can deploy cutting-edge diagnostics and personalized interventions sooner, not years after guidelines catch up.

The goal is straightforwardly bifold, even if the means are sophisticated—to help you become the strongest, sharpest, most resilient version of yourself now . . .and keep updating that version as you age.

Dr. Deep could dress that up in slogans, but underneath the language, that's what this model is about. Medicine is a relationship and a strategy now, not just a series of billables and quick symptom-checks.

If the current healthcare system is a fire department—vital when the house is burning but uninterested in your wiring the other 364 days of the year—then Velocity Health is closer to a personal architect and maintenance crew for the structure you live in. They're looking at the foundation, the load-bearing walls, the places where stress accumulates, and the systems you never notice until they fail.

That's why I say, without hesitation: **Dr. Deep's model is the future of healthcare.**

Not because it's trendy. Not because it has better branding. But because it actually aligns the incentives, the tools, and the time around the one thing that matters most in the long run:

Your healthspan as your ultimate asset.

A Ghostwriter's Challenge to You

As a ghostwriter, I usually stay invisible. My name might not be on the cover. My face won't be on the back jacket. I slip into the background so that the physician's voice can come through as clearly as possible.

Here, at the end of the book, I'm stepping briefly into the foreground to tell you something I've learned from sitting in this peculiar chair for this many years:

Most people underestimate how much their future self will thank them for one decisive season of seriousness. One season where you:

- Get the right diagnostics.

- Build the right team.

- Change the right habits.

- Stick with them long enough to see your lab numbers, your energy, your capacity, your mood fundamentally shift.

You don't need to live like a lab rat for the rest of

your life. You do need to stop living like your healthspan will somehow take care of itself.

You've just spent an entire book with a doctor who has shown you what is possible when you stop playing defense and start playing offense with your health. You've watched case studies of people who were you, in some form—overcommitted, overwhelmed, a little scared, a lot tired—who chose to step into a new way of doing healthcare. Now you get to decide if you're going to be one of them.

From my side of the page, I'll say this . . .

I've seen people write these books because they needed to justify selling another program.

I've seen people write these books because they were honest-to-God tired of watching patients slip through the cracks.

This is the second kind of book. This is the kind of book a doctor writes when he has seen enough to know the system won't fix itself and the only way forward is one patient, one practice, one family at a time choosing a different path.

You can't control every variable. But you can control whether you stay in a story where your health happens to you, or step into one where your healthspan is your ultimate asset—managed, protected, and grown on purpose.

It's your last window.

Take it.

Glossary

A1C

A blood test that measures your average blood sugar over the past two to three months. It's a key marker for prediabetes and diabetes risk and an early indicator of how well your body is handling glucose.

Advanced diagnostics

A deeper level of testing—beyond the usual basic labs and quick checkups—that includes imaging, expanded blood panels, genetic and epigenetic tests, and performance measures to reveal hidden risks long before disease shows up.

APOE

A gene involved in how your body handles cholesterol and fats. Certain APOE variants, like APOE4, are associated with a higher risk of Alzheimer's disease and cardiovascular problems, which can guide more personalized prevention strategies.

Apolipoprotein B (ApoB)

A blood marker that counts the number of "bad" cholesterol particles circulating in your blood. It's a more precise measure of cardiovascular risk than total cholesterol or LDL alone.

Ashramas

A traditional Hindu framework that divides life into

stages (student, householder, forest dweller, renunciate). This book uses it as a lens for understanding midlife purpose and how your mission evolves with age.

Biohacking

A do-it-yourself approach to health using gadgets, supplements, and quick fixes. In *The Ultimate Asset*, it's contrasted with deeper, physician-led care that focuses on systems, diagnostics, and long-term healthspan rather than short-term tricks.

Biomastery

The idea of mastering your biology through structured diagnostics, data-informed plans, and sustainable habits. I position this as the antidote to both burnout and shallow biohacking.

Biological age

An estimate of how "old" your body is functionally, based on markers like inflammation, metabolic health, fitness, and cognition. It can be younger or older than your calendar (chronological) age.

CAC (Coronary Artery Calcium) score

A CT-based scan that measures how much calcified plaque is in your coronary arteries. A higher CAC score means more plaque and a higher risk of heart attack, even if routine labs look "normal."

CCTA (Coronary CT Angiography)

An advanced CT scan that creates detailed images of your coronary arteries, showing both calcified and "soft" plaque. It helps reveal early heart disease risk and guides more aggressive prevention when needed.

CGM (Continuous Glucose Monitor)

A sensor you wear on your body that tracks blood sugar levels around the clock. It shows how your food, stress, sleep, and exercise affect your glucose in real time, making it easier to personalize your nutrition and lifestyle.

Concierge care

A membership-style medical model where you pay directly for more time, access, and personalized attention from your physician. It's the opposite of rushed, insurance-driven visits.

Concierge precision medicine

The combination of concierge access with data-driven, personalized care. In this book, it means a doctor who knows you well and uses advanced diagnostics to tailor your health plan to your unique biology and goals.

Constantia

A Latin term for steadiness or constancy. Along with *gravitas* and *humanitas*, it's used in the book to describe the mature virtues of later life—especially the reliability and groundedness people expect from elders.

Core Four

The four foundational pillars of health this book returns to repeatedly: sleep, nutrition, movement, and mental resilience. These are the collective base you must build before advanced diagnostics and therapies can truly pay off.

DEXA scan

A low-dose X-ray scan that measures bone density and body composition, including how much muscle and fat you have and where it's distributed. It's a key tool for understanding sarcopenia, visceral fat, and long-term metabolic risk.

Digital twin

A concept where a virtual model of your body and biology is created using data and simulations. Digital twins are a future direction for medicine, where treatment can be tested virtually before it's tried in real life.

Epigenetic age

A measure of how your environment and lifestyle have "marked" your genes over time, often estimated by specific DNA methylation patterns. Epigenetic age can move younger or older depending on how you live.

Epigenetics

The study of how lifestyle, environment, and experiences influence which genes are turned on or off without changing the DNA itself. This is a key idea behind why your future isn't fixed by genetics alone.

Executive health assessment

A comprehensive evaluation—often including advanced labs, imaging, and fitness tests—designed for high-achieving professionals. This book uses it as a model for how midlife adults can get a true picture of their health status.

Grandmother effect

A concept from evolutionary biology suggesting that grandparents—especially grandmothers—boost their grandchildren's survival and success. *The Ultimate Asset* uses it to illustrate why staying healthy into later decades matters for families and communities.

Gravitas

A Latin term for seriousness and moral weight. This book uses *gravitas* to describe the kind of presence and authority that healthy, purposeful elders can bring to their families, workplaces, and society.

Healthspan

The number of years you live in good health—with energy, capability, and clarity—rather than just the total number of years you're alive. It's the central "ultimate asset" this book teaches you to protect and extend.

Healthspan optimization

Intentionally shaping your lifestyle, diagnostics, and care so you extend your healthy, high-functioning years. It's the whole point of the Velocity Health model and the book's frameworks.

Homocysteine

An amino acid in the blood that, when elevated, is linked to higher risk of heart disease, stroke, and cognitive decline. This is a modifiable marker that can improve with targeted nutrition and lifestyle changes.

Humanitas

A Latin term for kindness and humane concern. Alongside *gravitas* and *constantia*, I use it in the book as part of the moral and emotional maturity we hope to grow into as we age.

Hyperbaric oxygen therapy (HBOT)

A treatment where you breathe pure oxygen in a pressurized chamber, increasing oxygen delivery to tissues. In my book, it appears as one of several advanced therapies to consider after foundations like sleep and nutrition are in place.

Ikigai

A Japanese concept meaning "a reason for being" or the intersection of what you love, what you're good at, what the world needs, and what you can be paid for. This book uses it when talking about purpose and midlife mission.

Insulin resistance

A state where your cells stop responding properly to insulin, forcing your pancreas to work harder to keep blood sugar in check. It's a major driver of metabolic syndrome and early cardiometabolic disease.

Mental resilience

Your capacity to handle stress, bounce back from setbacks, and maintain emotional stability. In the Core Four, it's treated as a trainable pillar, not just a personality trait.

Metabolic flexibility

Your body's ability to easily switch between burning carbohydrates and fats for fuel. Greater flexibility means better energy, easier fat loss, and more resilience under stress.

Metabolic health

The overall state of how well your body manages energy—blood sugar, blood pressure, lipids, and waist size. Good metabolic health supports a younger biological age and lower risk of chronic disease.

Metabolic syndrome

A cluster of conditions—such as high waist circumference, high blood pressure, elevated blood sugar, high triglycerides, and low HDL—that together increase your risk for heart disease, stroke, and diabetes.

Mitochondria

The "power plants" inside your cells that produce energy (ATP). This book references mitochondrial function as a core driver of energy, fatigue, and how old or young you feel day to day.

Peptides

Short chains of amino acids used as signaling molecules in the body. In my book, they appear as a category of advanced therapy that may enhance repair, recovery, or metabolic function when used carefully and strategically.

Precision medicine

An approach that tailors prevention and treatment to the individual using data—genes, labs, imaging, and lifestyle context—rather than one-size-fits-all guidelines.

PRP (Platelet-Rich Plasma)

A therapy where your own blood is spun down to concentrate platelets and growth factors, then injected into joints or tissues to promote healing. *The Ultimate*

Asset mentions PRP as one of several advanced interventions for the right patients.

Rapamycin

A drug that affects the mTOR pathway and is being studied for its potential longevity and healthspan benefits. In my book, it's part of the advanced therapeutics discussion—not a first-line tool, but a possible later lever.

Ren

A Confucian concept roughly meaning benevolence or human-heartedness. This book uses *ren* alongside other cultural frames to describe the mature, outward-focused purpose that often emerges in later life.

Sickcare

A critical term for the current healthcare system, which focuses on diagnosing and treating disease after it appears rather than preventing it. I contrast sickcare with proactive, healthspan-focused care.

Sleep hygiene

The set of habits and environmental choices—like light exposure, timing, temperature, and pre-bed routines—that strongly influence how well you sleep. It's a major lever in this book's sleep and recovery chapter.

Social determinants of health (SDOH)

Non-medical factors—such as housing, income, education, neighborhood, and social support—that heavily influence health outcomes. I reference SDOH when discussing why individual health choices exist inside larger systems and structures.

Testosterone replacement therapy (TRT)

Hormone therapy that boosts or replaces testosterone in people with clinically low levels. This book discusses TRT as a potential tool within a broader, carefully monitored hormonal and metabolic strategy.

Velocity Health Clinic

My concierge, precision medicine clinic, which serves as the living example of this book's philosophy—using advanced diagnostics, personalized plans, and ongoing support to extend healthspan.

VO$_2$ max

A measure of how much oxygen your body can use during intense exercise, often considered the gold standard of cardiovascular fitness. Higher VO$_2$ max is linked with lower mortality and a "younger" functional age.

Acknowledgments

To the love of my life Abigail, my beautiful children Devin and Lily, and to my extraordinary parents and family, whose unwavering love, patience, and support have sustained me through every challenge and triumph.

To the many mentors and colleagues across the healthcare field whose insight, guidance, and collaboration have profoundly shaped my thinking and practice.

To my patients, who have entrusted me with their care and, in doing so, allowed me to learn and grow alongside them. Their courage and commitment remain my greatest teachers.

To my writing partner, Joshua Lisec, whose extraordinary talent helped me give shape and voice to ideas that had long lived only in my head. Through his partnership, I have been able to communicate my message far beyond the walls of my clinic and begin to build a lasting legacy. Thank you, also, for contributing the afterword—and under your own name.

To my team, Morgan, Brock, and the entire early family at Velocity who pour their heart and soul into improving lives every day. To my business partners and early investors, whose belief in me and in the vision for Velocity Health Clinic transformed possibility into reality. Without their faith and support, this journey would not have been possible.

About the Author

Dr. Sandeep "Deep" Palakodeti brings over two decades of experience at the intersection of value-based care, longevity medicine, and healthcare innovation. As the Founder and CEO of Velocity Health, Dr. Deep is focused on building next-generation models of care that prioritize prevention, personalization, and long-term wellness.

He earned both his Doctor of Medicine (MD) and Master of Public Health (MPH) degrees from Wright State University. He went on to complete his Internal Medicine residency at Kaiser Permanente, one of the nation's most respected integrated healthcare systems. He then was accepted into a prestigious fellowship in Healthcare Innovation at Harvard Medical School, where he deepened his expertise in designing scalable, patient-centered healthcare solutions.

Throughout his career, Dr. Palakodeti has held clinical and executive roles across renowned institutions, including the Mayo Clinic and CareMore Health. He has also served in leadership positions within health tech startups and major academic medical centers, consistently working at the forefront of care model redesign and digital health integration.

Dr. Deep is recognized for his forward-thinking leadership and commitment to improving population health outcomes through data-driven, holistic approaches to medicine.

Learn more at www.velocityhealthclinic.com.

Endnotes

1 Jasninder S. Dhaliwal and Ashujot Kaur Dang, "Reducing Hospital Readmissions," in StatPearls (Treasure Island, FL: StatPearls Publishing, 2024), last modified June 7, 2024, https://www.ncbi.nlm.nih.gov/books/NBK606114/.

2 Kenneth Mubiru. "The Life of an African Elephant Matriarch: The Mother and the Leader." J.T Safaris, November 12, 2024. https://jtsafarisug.com/2024/11/12/the-life-of-an-african-elephant-matriarch-the-mother-and-the-leader.

3 Karen McComb et al., "Leadership in Elephants: The Adaptive Value of Age," Proceedings of the Royal Society B: Biological Sciences 278, no. 1722 (2011): 3270-76, https://doi.org/10.1098/rspb.2011.0168.

4 Lauren J.N. Brent et al., "Ecological Knowledge, Leadership, and the Evolution of Menopause in Killer Whales," Current Biology 25, no. 6 (2015): 746-750, https://doi.org/10.1016/j.cub.2015.01.037.

5 Living with Wolves. "The Social Wolf." https://www.livingwithwolves.org/about-wolves/social-wolf/.

6 Robin Marantz Henig, "Reveling in the Grandmother Hypothesis," Cusp (blog), Psychology Today, October 29, 2015, https://www.psychologytoday.com/us/blog/cusp/201510/reveling-in-the-grandmother-hypothesis.

7 Henig, "Reveling in the Grandmother Hypothesis."

8 James G. Herndon, "The Grandmother Effect: Implications for Studies on Aging and Cognition," Gerontology 56, no. 1 (2010): 73-79, https://doi.org/10.1159/000236045.

9   Mat McDermott, "What Are the Four Stages of Hindu Life?," Hindu American Foundation, January 13, 2017, https://www.hinduamerican.org/blog/what-are-the-four-stages-of-hindu-life/.

10   JKYog Team, "Duty vs Desire: What Shree Krishna Taught Arjuna About Moral Dilemmas," Swami Mukundananda Blog (blog), August 2, 2025, https://www.jkyog.org/blog/duty-vs-desire-krishna-on-moral-dilemmas.

11   John Messerly, "Summary of Cicero, 'On Old Age,'" Reason and Meaning, August 28, 2017, https://reasonandmeaning.com/2017/08/28/summary-of-cicero-on-aging/.

12   https://www.otterbein.edu/alumni/wp-content/uploads/sites/4/2020/11/Selections-from-Confucius-Analects.pdf

13   Calm Editorial Team, "Ikigai: What It Is and How to Use Ikigai to Find Your Purpose," Calm Blog, December 7, 2023, https://www.calm.com/blog/ikigai.

14   "The Role of Native American Women in Plains Tribes," Wind River Country, March 13, 2023, https://windriver.org/the-womens-role/.

15   Allen Johnson, "How to Say Grandma in Navajo: Honoring the Elderly in Indigenous Language," The Techy Life, June 7, 2024, https://thetechy.life/how-to-say-grandma-in-navajo/.

16   D. L. Birchfield, "Sioux," Countries and Their Cultures, The Gale Group Inc., 2008, https://www.everyculture.com/multi/Pa-Sp/Sioux.html.

17   Guy Gibbon, "Sioux," in Encyclopedia of the Great Plains, ed. David J. Wishart (Lincoln: University of Nebraska Press, 2011), https://plainshumanities.unl.edu/encyclopedia/doc/egp.na.107.html.

18   Paul Boyer, "Young and Old Alike: Children and the
        Elderly Are a Priority in Native American Cultures,"
        Tribal College Journal of American Indian Higher
        Education, February 15, 1992, https://tribalcollege-
        journal.org/young-alike-children-elderly-priority-na-
        tive-american-cultures/.

19   Ultimate Care, "How Often Should Grandparents See
        Their Grandchildren," Ultimate Care NY, March 14,
        2025, https://www.ultimatecareny.com/resources/how-
        often-should-grandparents-see-their-grandchildren.

20   Usama Khan, "River Cruise Statistics: Key Trends
        for 2025," Retirement Living, November 14, 2025,
        https://www.retirementliving.com/best-river-cruises/
        river-cruise-statistics.

21   Taylor Bowley, Luxury Is Back in Fashion?, Consum-
        er Morsel (Bank of America Institute, January 28,
        2025), https://institute.bankofamerica.com/content/
        dam/economic-insights/luxury-spending.pdf.

22   National Association of Realtors, "Baby Boomers
        Regain Top Spot as Largest Share of Home Buyers,"
        April 1, 2025, https://www.nar.realtor/newsroom/
        baby-boomers-regain-top-spot-as-largest-share-of-
        home-buyers.

23   National Association of Realtors, "Baby Boomers
        Regain Top Spot."

24   "I'm Spending All of My Kids' Inheritance Money: 'En-
        titled' Gen Zers Shouldn't Expect Anything," New York
        Post, July 15, 2024, https://nypost.com/2024/07/15/life-
        style/im-spending-all-of-my-kids-inheritance-money-
        entitled-gen-zers-shouldnt-expect-anything/.

25   "Why Spending Your Kids' Inheritance Can Make
        Sense," Become Wealth, accessed December 18, 2025,
        https://www.become.nz/articles/5-reasons-why-you-
        should-spend-your-kids-inheritance.

26   "Simon Cowell's Decision about Son Eric Not In-
        heriting $600M Fortune Sparks Debate," The Express
        Tribune, October 31, 2025, https://tribune.com.pk/
        story/2575131/simon-cowells-decision-about-son-eric-
        not-inheriting-600m-fortune-sparks-debate.

27   Simon Sinek, "How Great Leaders Inspire Action,"
        TED, May 4, 2010, YouTube video, 17:47, https://www.
        youtube.com/watch?v=qp0HIF3SfI4.

28   Patrick L. Hill and Nicholas A. Turiano, "Purpose in
        Life as a Predictor of Mortality across Adulthood," Psy-
        chological Science 25, no. 7 (2014): 1482-86, https://doi.
        org/10.1177/0956797614531799.

29   "How Sleep Affects Your Health," National Heart, Lung,
        and Blood Institute, last modified June 15, 2022, https://
        www.nhlbi.nih.gov/health/sleep-deprivation/health-ef-
        fects.

30   Claire Caruso and Roger R. Rosa, "Sleep and Work,"
        NIOSH Science Blog (blog), Centers for Disease Control
        and Prevention, March 8, 2012, last modified No-
        vember 25, 2024, https://blogs.cdc.gov/niosh-science-
        blog/2012/03/08/sleep-and-work/.

31   Kristen Harknett, Daniel Schneider, and Rebecca Wolfe,
        "Losing Sleep over Work Scheduling? The Relationship
        between Work Schedules and Sleep Quality for Service
        Sector Workers," SSM - Population Health 12 (2020):
        100681, https://doi.org/10.1016/j.ssmph.2020.100681.

32   Brian G. Arndt et al., "Tethered to the EHR: Primary
        Care Physician Workload Assessment Using EHR Event
        Log Data and Time-Motion Observations," The Annals
        of Family Medicine 15, no. 5 (2017): 419-26, https://doi.
        org/10.1370/afm.2121.

33   Sheikh Bilal Ahmad et al., "Melatonin and Health:
        Insights of Melatonin Action, Biological Functions, and
        Associated Disorders," Cellular and Molecular Neurobi-
        ology 43, no. 6 (2023): 2437-58, https://doi.org/10.1007/
        s10571-023-01324-w.

34   Ahmad et al., "Melatonin and Health," 2440.

35   Carolin Franziska Reichert, Tom Deboer, and Hans-Pe-
      ter Landolt, "Adenosine, Caffeine, and Sleep-Wake Reg-
      ulation: State of the Science and Perspectives," Journal
      of Sleep Research 31, no. 4 (2022): e13597, https://doi.
      org/10.1111/jsr.13597.

36   Reichert, Deboer, and Landolt, "Adenosine, Caffeine,
      and Sleep-Wake Regulation," e13597.

37   Reichert, Deboer, and Landolt, "Adenosine, Caffeine,
      and Sleep-Wake Regulation," e13597.

38   Reichert, Deboer, and Landolt, "Adenosine, Caffeine,
      and Sleep-Wake Regulation," e13597.

39   Nor Amira Syahira Mohd Azmi et al., "Cortisol on
      Circadian Rhythm and Its Effect on Cardiovascular Sys-
      tem," International Journal of Environmental Research
      and Public Health 18, no. 2 (2021): 676, https://doi.
      org/10.3390/ijerph18020676.

40   Nicole P. Bowles et al., "The Circadian System Mod-
      ulates the Cortisol Awakening Response in Humans,"
      Frontiers in Neuroscience 16 (2022), https://doi.
      org/10.3389/fnins.2022.995452.

41   Nicholas C. Nicolaides et al., "HPA Axis and Sleep," in
      Endotext, ed. Kenneth R. Feingold et al. (MDText.com,
      2000-), last modified November 24, 2020, https://www.
      ncbi.nlm.nih.gov/books/NBK279071/.

42   Sarnataro, R., Velasco, C.D., Monaco, N. et al. Mito-
      chondrial origins of the pressure to sleep. Nature 645,
      722-728 (2025). https://doi.org/10.1038/s41586-025-
      09261-y

43   Nicolaides et al., "HPA Axis and Sleep."

44   Nicolaides et al., "HPA Axis and Sleep."

45   Christine Blume et al., "Melatonin Suppression Does Not Automatically Alter Sleepiness, Vigilance, Sensory Processing, or Sleep," Sleep 45, no. 11 (2022): zsac199, https://doi.org/10.1093/sleep/zsac199.

46   Joshua J. Gooley et al., "Exposure to Room Light before Bedtime Suppresses Melatonin Onset and Shortens Melatonin Duration in Humans," Journal of Clinical Endocrinology and Metabolism 96, no. 3 (2011): E463, https://doi.org/10.1210/jc.2010-2098.

47   Tianyi Huang, Sara Mariani, and Susan Redline, "Sleep Irregularity and Risk of Cardiovascular Events: The Multi-Ethnic Study of Atherosclerosis," Journal of the American College of Cardiology 75, no. 9 (2020): 991-999, https://doi.org/10.1016/j.jacc.2019.12.054.

48   Brett A. Messman et al., "Irregular Sleep Is Linked to Poorer Mental Health: A Pooled Analysis of Eight Studies," Sleep Health 10, no. 4 (2024): 493-99, https://doi.org/10.1016/j.sleh.2024.03.004.

49   Andrew J. K. Phillips et al., "Irregular Sleep/Wake Patterns Are Associated with Poorer Academic Performance and Delayed Circadian and Sleep/Wake Timing," Scientific Reports 7, no. 1 (2017): 3216, https://doi.org/10.1038/s41598-017-03171-4.

50   Samuel E. Jones et al., "Genome-Wide Association Analyses of Chronotype in 697,828 Individuals Provides Insights into Circadian Rhythms," Nature Communications 10, no. 1 (2019): 343, https://doi.org/10.1038/s41467-018-08259-7.

51   Marc Wittmann, Jenny Dinich, Martha Merrow, and Till Roenneberg, "Social Jetlag: Misalignment of Biological and Social Time," Chronobiology International 23, no. 1-2 (2006): 497-509, https://doi.org/10.1080/07420520500545979.

52   Haowen Zou, Hongliang Zhou, Rui Yan, Zhijian Yao,
        and Qing Lu, "Chronotype, Circadian Rhythm, and
        Psychiatric Disorders: Recent Evidence and Potential
        Mechanisms," Frontiers in Neuroscience 16 (2022),
        https://doi.org/10.3389/fnins.2022.811771.

53   Patricia M. Wong et al., "Social Jetlag, Chronotype, and
        Cardiometabolic Risk," The Journal of Clinical Endo-
        crinology & Metabolism 100, no. 12 (2015): 4612-4620,
        https://doi.org/10.1210/jc.2015-2923.

54   Marc Wittmann, Jenny Dinich, Martha Merrow,
        and Till Roenneberg, "Social Jetlag: Misalignment
        of Biological and Social Time," Chronobiology In-
        ternational 23, no. 1-2 (2006): 497, https://doi.
        org/10.1080/07420520500545979.

55   Kurt Kräuchi, Christian Cajochen, Esther Werth, and
        Anna Wirz-Justice, "Functional Link between Distal Va-
        sodilation and Sleep-Onset Latency?," American Journal
        of Physiology-Regulatory, Integrative and Comparative
        Physiology 278, no. 3 (2000): R741-R748, https://doi.
        org/10.1152/ajpregu.2000.278.3.R741.

56   Shahab Haghayegh et al., "Before-Bedtime Passive Body
        Heating by Warm Shower or Bath to Improve Sleep: A
        Systematic Review and Meta-Analysis," Sleep Medicine
        Reviews 46 (2019): 124-35, https://doi.org/10.1016/j.
        smrv.2019.04.008.

57   Kurt Kräuchi and Anna Wirz-Justice, "Circadian Clues
        to Sleep Onset Mechanisms," Neuropsychopharmacol-
        ogy 25, S1 (2001): S92-S96, https://doi.org/10.1016/
        S0893-133X(01)00315-3.

58   Yelin Ko and Joo-Young Lee, "Effects of Feet Warming
        Using Bed Socks on Sleep Quality and Thermoregu-
        latory Responses in a Cool Environment," Journal of
        Physiological Anthropology 37, no. 1 (2018): 13, https://
        doi.org/10.1186/s40101-018-0172-z.

59   Cleveland Clinic, "What's the Best Temperature for Sleep?" Health Essentials, November 16, 2021, https://health.clevelandclinic.org/what-is-the-ideal-sleeping-temperature-for-my-bedroom.

60   Robert R. Freedman, "Menopausal Hot Flashes: Mechanisms, Endocrinology, Treatment," The Journal of Steroid Biochemistry and Molecular Biology 142 (2014): 115-120, https://doi.org/10.1016/j.jsbmb.2013.08.010.

61   Nancy E. Avis, Beverly J. Levine, and Remy Coeytaux, "Results of a Pilot Study of a Cooling Mattress Pad to Reduce Vasomotor Symptoms and Improve Sleep," Menopause 29, no. 8 (2022): 973-78, https://doi.org/10.1097/GME.0000000000002010.

62   Andrew Huberman, "Dr. Matt Walker: The Biology of Sleep & Your Unique Sleep Needs | Huberman Lab Guest Series," April 3, 2024, YouTube video, 2:59:33, https://www.youtube.com/watch?v=-OBCwiPPfEU.

63   Michael H. Bonnet and Donna L. Arand, "Hyperarousal and Insomnia: State of the Science," Sleep Medicine Reviews 14, no. 1 (2010): 9-15, https://doi.org/10.1016/j.smrv.2009.05.002.

64   Ravindra P. Nagendra, Nirmala Maruthai, and Bindu M. Kutty, "Meditation and Its Regulatory Role on Sleep," Frontiers in Neurology 3 (2012): 54, https://doi.org/10.3389/fneur.2012.00054.

65   Valērija Steinmane and Andra Fernate, "The Effect of Breathing Exercises on Adults' Sleep Quality: An Intervention That Works," Frontiers in Sleep 4 (2025), https://doi.org/10.3389/frsle.2025.1603713.

66   Darian Dozier, "How Warm Baths Impact Sleep: The Science of Soaking for Better Rest," AncSleep Blog, Anchorage Sleep Center, May 13, 2025, https://info.ancsleep.com/blog/how-warm-baths-impact-sleep-the-science-of-soaking-for-better-rest.

67   Rachel Leproult et al., "Transition from Dim to Bright Light in the Morning Induces an Immediate Elevation of Cortisol Levels," The Journal of Clinical Endocrinology & Metabolism 86, no. 1 (2001): 151, https://doi.org/10.1210/jcem.86.1.7102.

68   Isabella Robertson-Dixon et al., "The Influence of Light Wavelength on Human HPA Axis Rhythms: A Systematic Review," Life 13, no. 10 (2023): 1968, https://doi.org/10.3390/life13101968.

69   Joshua J. Gooley et al., "Exposure to Room Light before Bedtime Suppresses Melatonin Onset and Shortens Melatonin Duration in Humans," The Journal of Clinical Endocrinology & Metabolism 96, no. 3 (2011): E463-E472, https://doi.org/10.1210/jc.2010-2098.

70   Ivy C. Mason et al., "Light Exposure during Sleep Impairs Cardiometabolic Function," Proceedings of the National Academy of Sciences 119, no. 12 (2022): e2113290119, https://doi.org/10.1073/pnas.2113290119.

71   Esther Donga et al., "A Single Night of Partial Sleep Deprivation Induces Insulin Resistance in Multiple Metabolic Pathways in Healthy Subjects," The Journal of Clinical Endocrinology & Metabolism 95, no. 6 (2010): 2963-68, https://doi.org/10.1210/jc.2009-2430.

72   Yingting Cao et al., "Dinner Fat Intake and Sleep Duration and Self-Reported Sleep Parameters over Five Years: Findings from the Jiangsu Nutrition Study of Chinese Adults," Nutrition 32, no. 9 (September 2016): 970-74, https://doi.org/10.1016/j.nut.2016.02.012.

73   "Better Sleep: 3 Simple Diet Tweaks," Johns Hopkins Medicine, accessed December 20, 2025, https://www.hopkinsmedicine.org/health/wellness-and-prevention/better-sleep-3-simple-diet-tweaks.

74   Steven B. Roach, "Wake up at 3 a.m. and Can't Fall Back Asleep? Consider Low Blood Sugar," Carolinas Thyroid Institute, October 23, 2012, https://www.carolinasthyroidinstitute.com/wake-up-at-3-a-m-and-cant-fall-back-asleep-consider-low-blood-sugar/.

75   David Benton, Anthony Bloxham, Chantelle Gaylor, Anthony Brennan, and Hayley A. Young, "Carbohydrate and Sleep: An Evaluation of Putative Mechanisms," Frontiers in Nutrition 9 (2022), https://doi.org/10.3389/fnut.2022.933898.

76   Bonnie Spring, "Recent Research on the Behavioral Effects of Tryptophan and Carbohydrate," Nutrition and Health 3, no. 1-2 (1984): 55-67, https://doi.org/10.1177/026010608400300204.

77   Benton et al., "Carbohydrate and Sleep."

78   Reichert, Deboer, and Landolt, "Adenosine, Caffeine, and Sleep-Wake Regulation," e13597.

79   Christopher Drake, Timothy Roehrs, John Shambroom, and Thomas Roth, "Caffeine Effects on Sleep Taken 0, 3, or 6 Hours before Going to Bed," Journal of Clinical Sleep Medicine 9, no. 11 (2013): 1195-, https://doi.org/10.5664/jcsm.3170.

80   Calm Editorial Team, "Does Alcohol Affect REM Sleep? Here's What to Know and How to Fix It," Calm Blog, June 20, 2024, https://www.calm.com/blog/alcohol-rem-sleep.

81   Chaoran Ma et al., "Alcohol Consumption and Probable Rapid Eye Movement Sleep Behavior Disorder," Annals of Clinical and Translational Neurology 5, no. 10 (2018): 1176-1183, https://doi.org/10.1002/acn3.630.

82   Ibrahim Sönmez et al., "Unmasking Obstructive Sleep Apnea: Estimated Prevalence and Impact in the United States," Respiratory Medicine 248 (2025): 108348, https://doi.org/10.1016/j.rmed.2025.108348.

83   Edward O. Bixler, Alexandros N. Vgontzas, Thomas Ten Have, Kathy Tyson, and Anthony Kales, "Effects of Age on Sleep Apnea in Men: I. Prevalence and Severity," American Journal of Respiratory and Critical Care Medicine 157, no. 1 (1997): 144-48, https://doi.org/10.1164/ajrccm.157.1.9706079.

84   Jatuporn Wanchaitanawong et al., "Obstructive Sleep Apnea Detection and Prevalence in Men and Women Using a Continuous Large U.S. Sample by Home Under-Mattress Devices," Sleep Medicine 136 (2025): 106808, https://doi.org/10.1016/j.sleep.2025.106808.

85   H. A. McLean et al., "Effect of Treating Severe Nasal Obstruction on the Severity of Obstructive Sleep Apnoea," European Respiratory Journal 25, no. 3 (2005): 521-27, https://doi.org/10.1183/09031936.05.00045004.

86   Terry Young, Larel Finn, and Hyon Kim, "Nasal Obstruction as a Risk Factor for Sleep-Disordered Breathing," Journal of Allergy and Clinical Immunology 99, no. 2 (1997): S757-62, https://doi.org/10.1016/S0091-6749(97)70124-6.

87   Yuanyuan Li, Yanli Hao, Fang Fan, and Bin Zhang, "The Role of Microbiome in Insomnia, Circadian Disturbance and Depression," Frontiers in Psychiatry 9 (2018): 669, https://doi.org/10.3389/fpsyt.2018.00669.

88   Monika Sejbuk, Adam Siebieszuk, and Anna Maria Witkowska, "The Role of Gut Microbiome in Sleep Quality and Health: Dietary Strategies for Microbiota Support," Nutrients 16, no. 14 (2024): 2259, https://doi.org/10.3390/nu16142259.

89   Sejbuk, Siebieszuk, and Witkowska, "Role of Gut Microbiome," 2259.

90   Malka N. Halgamuge, "Pineal Melatonin Level Disruption in Humans Due to Electromagnetic Fields and IC-NIRP Limits," Radiation Protection Dosimetry 154, no. 4 (2013): 405-416, https://doi.org/10.1093/rpd/ncs255.

91   Reto Huber et al., "Exposure to Pulsed High-Frequency Electromagnetic Field during Waking Affects Human Sleep EEG," NeuroReport 11, no. 15 (2000): 3321-3325, https://doi.org/10.1097/00001756-200010200-00012.

92   Daniel Noyed, "How Electronics Affect Sleep," Sleep Foundation, last modified July 10, 2025, https://www.sleepfoundation.org/how-sleep-works/how-electronics-affect-sleep.

93   Jean-Philippe Chaput et al., "Sleep Timing, Sleep Consistency, and Health in Adults: A Systematic Review," Applied Physiology, Nutrition, and Metabolism 45, no. 10 (Suppl. 2) (2020): S232-S247, https://doi.org/10.1139/apnm-2020-0032.

94   Angela S. Lillehei et al., "Effect of Inhaled Lavender and Sleep Hygiene on Self-Reported Sleep Issues: A Randomized Controlled Trial," Journal of Alternative and Complementary Medicine 21, no. 7 (2015): 430-438, https://doi.org/10.1089/acm.2014.0327.

95   Sian Ferguson, "Does ASMR Help You Sleep? Research, Benefits, Tips," Healthline, April 10, 2025, https://www.healthline.com/health/does-asmr-help-you-sleep.

96   Shun-Ping Hu et al., "Effect of Sleep Ambient Music on Sleep Quality and Mental Health in College Students: A Self-Controlled Study," Frontiers in Psychology 14 (2023), https://doi.org/10.3389/fpsyg.2023.1171939.

97   Rachel R. Markwald, Imran Iftikhar, and Shawn D. Youngstedt, "Behavioral Strategies, Including Exercise, for Addressing Insomnia," ACSM's Health & Fitness Journal 22, no. 2 (2018): 23-29, https://doi.org/10.1249/FIT.0000000000000375.

98   Norman J. Temple, "The Origins of the Obesity Epidemic in the USA–Lessons for Today," Nutrients 14, no. 20 (2022): 4253, https://doi.org/10.3390/nu14204253.

99   Temple, "Origins of the Obesity Epidemic," 4253.

100   Donald J. McNamara, "The Fifty Year Rehabilitation of the Egg," Nutrients 7, no. 10 (2015): 8716-8722, https://doi.org/10.3390/nu7105429.

101   Frédéric Leroy and Nathan Cofnas, "Should Dietary Guidelines Recommend Low Red Meat Intake?," Critical Reviews in Food Science and Nutrition 60, no. 16 (2020): 2763-72, https://doi.org/10.1080/10408398.2019.1657063.

102   Lee S. Gross et al., "Increased Consumption of Refined Carbohydrates and the Epidemic of Type 2 Diabetes in the United States: An Ecologic Assessment," The American Journal of Clinical Nutrition 79, no. 5 (2004): 774-779, https://doi.org/10.1093/ajcn/79.5.774.

103   Frank B. Hu, "Are Refined Carbohydrates Worse than Saturated Fat?," The American Journal of Clinical Nutrition 91, no. 6 (2010): 1541-1542, https://doi.org/10.3945/ajcn.2010.29622.

104   Michele N. Ravelli and Dale A. Schoeller, "Traditional Self-Reported Dietary Instruments Are Prone to Inaccuracies and New Approaches Are Needed," Frontiers in Nutrition 7 (2020): 90, https://doi.org/10.3389/fnut.2020.00090.

105   Pauli Ohukainen, Jyrki K. Virtanen, and Mika Ala-Korpela, "Vexed Causal Inferences in Nutritional Epidemiology—Call for Genetic Help," International Journal of Epidemiology 51, no. 1 (2022): 6, https://doi.org/10.1093/ije/dyab152.

106   Valeria Tosti, Beatrice Bertozzi, and Luigi Fontana, "Health Benefits of the Mediterranean Diet: Metabolic and Molecular Mechanisms," The Journals of Gerontology: Series A 73, no. 3 (2018): 318-326, https://doi.org/10.1093/gerona/glx227.

107   Alison McCook, "Errors Trigger Retraction of Study on Mediterranean Diet's Heart Benefits," NPR, June 13, 2018, https://www.npr.org/sections/health-shots/2018/06/13/619619302/errors-trigger-retraction-of-study-on-mediterranean-diets-heart-benefits.

108   Sharon F. Daley et al., "The Ketogenic Diet: Clinical
        Applications, Evidence-based Indications, and Imple-
        mentation," in StatPearls (Treasure Island, FL: StatPearls
        Publishing, 2023), last modified December 13, 2025.
        https://www.ncbi.nlm.nih.gov/books/NBK499830/.

109   Jennifer T. Batch et al., "Advantages and Disadvantages
        of the Ketogenic Diet: A Review Article," Cureus 12, no.
        8 (2020): e9639, https://doi.org/10.7759/cureus.9639.

110   Ehsan Ghaedi et al., "Effects of a Paleolithic Diet on
        Cardiovascular Disease Risk Factors: A Systematic
        Review and Meta-Analysis of Randomized Controlled
        Trials," Advances in Nutrition 10, no. 4 (2019): 634-46,
        https://doi.org/10.1093/advances/nmz007.

111   "Is the Paleo Diet Healthy? It's Complicated," Harvard
        T.H. Chan School of Public Health, November 18, 2020,
        https://hsph.harvard.edu/news/paleo-diet-health-bene-
        fits-complicated/.

112   Emily Moskal, "Twin Research Indicates That a Vegan
        Diet Improves Cardiovascular Health," Stanford Med-
        icine, November 30, 2023, https://med.stanford.edu/
        news/all-news/2023/11/twin-diet-vegan-cardiovascular.
        html.

113   Anna R. Ogilvie et al., "Fracture Risk in Vegetarians
        and Vegans: The Role of Diet and Metabolic Factors,"
        Current Osteoporosis Reports 20, no. 6 (2022): 442-52,
        https://doi.org/10.1007/s11914-022-00754-7.

114   Nana Chung et al., "Non-exercise Activity Thermo-
        genesis (NEAT): A Component of Total Daily Energy
        Expenditure," Journal of Exercise Nutrition & Biochem-
        istry 22, no. 2 (2018): 23-30, https://doi.org/10.20463/
        jenb.2018.0013.

115   James A. Levine et al., "Non-Exercise Activity Ther-
        mogenesis: The Crouching Tiger Hidden Dragon of
        Societal Weight Gain," Arteriosclerosis, Thrombosis,
        and Vascular Biology 26, no. 4 (2006): 729, https://doi.
        org/10.1161/01.ATV.0000205848.83210.73.

116   Bernard M. F. M. Duvivier et al., "Minimal Intensity
       Physical Activity (Standing and Walking) of Longer Du-
       ration Improves Insulin Action and Plasma Lipids More
       than Shorter Periods of Moderate to Vigorous Exercise
       (Cycling) in Sedentary Subjects When Energy Expendi-
       ture Is Comparable," PLOS ONE 8, no. 2 (2013): e55542,
       https://doi.org/10.1371/journal.pone.0055542.

117   Johnston CS, Kim CM, Buller AJ. Vinegar improves in-
       sulin sensitivity to a high-carbohydrate meal in subjects
       with insulin resistance or type 2 diabetes. Diabetes Care.
       2004 Jan;27(1):281-2. doi: 10.2337/diacare.27.1.281.
       PMID: 14694010.

118   Panayota Mitrou et al., "Vinegar Consumption Increas-
       es Insulin-Stimulated Glucose Uptake by the Forearm
       Muscle in Humans with Type 2 Diabetes," Journal of
       Diabetes Research 2015 (2015): 175204, https://doi.
       org/10.1155/2015/175204.

119   Mitrou et al., "Vinegar Consumption."

120   Stephen J. Simpson et al., "Weight Gain during the
       Menopause Transition: Evidence for a Mechanism De-
       pendent on Protein Leverage," BJOG: An International
       Journal of Obstetrics & Gynaecology 130, no. 1 (2023):
       4-10, https://doi.org/10.1111/1471-0528.17290.

121   Simpson et al., "Weight Gain during the Menopause
       Transition," 4.

122   Margrit Richter et al., "Revised Reference Values
       for the Intake of Protein," Annals of Nutrition and
       Metabolism 74, no. 3 (2019): 242-250, https://doi.
       org/10.1159/000499374.

123   Travis B. Conley et al., "Age and Sex Affect Protein
       Metabolism at Protein Intakes That Span the Range of
       Adequacy: Comparison of Leucine Kinetics and Nitro-
       gen Balance Data," The Journal of Nutritional Biochem-
       istry 24, no. 4 (2013): 693, https://doi.org/10.1016/j.
       jnutbio.2012.03.021.

124   Dangzhen Liu et al., "Efficacy and Safety of Berber-
        ine on the Components of Metabolic Syndrome: A
        Systematic Review and Meta-Analysis of Randomized
        Placebo-Controlled Trials," Frontiers in Pharma-
        cology 16 (2025): 1572197, https://doi.org/10.3389/
        fphar.2025.1572197.

125   Yunqi Weng et al., "Nattokinase: An Oral Antithrom-
        botic Agent for the Prevention of Cardiovascular
        Disease," International Journal of Molecular Sciences 18,
        no. 3 (2017): 523, https://doi.org/10.3390/ijms18030523.

126   Weng et al., "Nattokinase," 523.

127   Quagliani D, Felt-Gunderson P. Closing America's
        Fiber Intake Gap: Communication Strategies From a
        Food and Fiber Summit. Am J Lifestyle Med. 2016 Jul
        7;11(1):80-85. doi: 10.1177/1559827615588079. PMID:
        30202317; PMCID: PMC6124841.

128   Kellen V. Lambeau and Johnson W. McRorie Jr., "Fiber
        Supplements and Clinically Proven Health Benefits:
        How to Recognize and Recommend an Effective Fiber
        Therapy," Journal of the American Association of Nurse
        Practitioners 29, no. 4 (2017): 216-23, https://doi.
        org/10.1002/2327-6924.12447.

129   Andrea N. Giancoli, "Fiber: Update on Fiber Sup-
        plements — What Dietitians Need to Know," Today's
        Dietitian 19, no. 2 (2017): 10, https://www.todaysdieti-
        tian.com/fiber-update-on-fiber-supplements-what-di-
        etitians-need-to-know/.

130   Giancoli, "Fiber: Update on Fiber Supplements," 10.

131   Todd B. Bates, "High-Fiber Foods May Boost Gut Bac-
        teria to Control Diabetes," Rutgers University, March 28,
        2018, https://www.rutgers.edu/news/high-fiber-foods-
        may-boost-gut-bacteria-control-diabetes.

132   Alice van der Schoot et al., "The Effect of Fiber Sup-
       plementation on Chronic Constipation in Adults: An
       Updated Systematic Review and Meta-Analysis of
       Randomized Controlled Trials," The American Journal
       of Clinical Nutrition 116, no. 4 (2022): 953-969, https://
       doi.org/10.1093/ajcn/nqac184.

133   Eliana Bistriche Giuntini, Fabiana Andrea Hoffmann Sardá,
       and Elizabete Wenzel de Menezes, "The Effects of Soluble
       Dietary Fibers on Glycemic Response: An Overview and
       Futures Perspectives," Foods 11, no. 23 (2022): 3934, https://
       doi.org/10.3390/foods11233934.

134   Layla A. Alahmari, "Dietary Fiber Influence on Overall
       Health, with an Emphasis on CVD, Diabetes, Obesity,
       Colon Cancer, and Inflammation," Frontiers in Nu-
       trition 11 (2024): 1510564, https://doi.org/10.3389/
       fnut.2024.1510564.

135   Cindy Crawford et al., "Analysis of Select Dietary
       Supplement Products Marketed to Support or Boost the
       Immune System," JAMA Network Open 5, no. 8 (2022):
       e2226040, https://doi.org/10.1001/jamanetworko-
       pen.2022.26040.

136   United States Pharmacopeial Convention, "USP Veri-
       fied Mark," USP, accessed December 21, 2025, https://
       www.usp.org/verification-services/verified-mark.

137   https://www.nsf.org/consumer-resources/articles/cer-
       tified-for-sport-program"Certified for Sport® Program,"
       NSF, accessed December 21, 2024, https://www.nsf.org/
       consumer-resources/articles/certified-for-sport-pro-
       gram.

138   U.S. Food and Drug Administration, "FDA 101: Dietary
       Supplements," June 2, 2022, https://www.fda.gov/con-
       sumers/consumer-updates/fda-101-dietary-supple-
       ments.

139   Jeff Chen, "Physician Scientist: Consumers Beware: Most Supplements Lack Proof," Newsweek, April 18, 2023, https://www.newsweek.com/physician-scientist-consumers-beware-most-supplements-lack-proof-1794814.

140   Ekaterina Galkina Cleary et al., "Contribution of NIH Funding to New Drug Approvals 2010–2016," Proceedings of the National Academy of Sciences of the United States of America 115, no. 10 (2018): 2329-34, https://doi.org/10.1073/pnas.1715368115.

141   Jeffrey Millstein, "The Truth About Supplements: 5 Things You Should Know," Penn Medicine Health and Wellness Blog, February 2020, archived March 31, 2020, at the Wayback Machine, https://web.archive.org/web/20200331043530/https://www.pennmedicine.org/updates/blogs/health-and-wellness/2020/february/the-truth-about-supplements.

142   Josh Davis, "Is 'Zone 2' Cardio the Best for Your Health?," Houston Methodist, October 16, 2025, https://www.houstonmethodist.org/blog/articles/2025/oct/is-zone-2-cardio-the-best-for-your-health/.

143   Davis, "Is 'Zone 2' Cardio."

144   Wayne L. Westcott, "Resistance Training Is Medicine: Effects of Strength Training on Health," Current Sports Medicine Reports 11, no. 4 (2012): 209-216, https://doi.org/10.1249/JSR.0b013e31825dabb8.

145   El Camino Health, "More than Muscle Mass: Benefits of Strength Training," November 2024, https://www.elcaminohealth.org/stay-healthy/blog/more-than-muscle-mass.

146   Yahai Wang et al., "Low Skeletal Muscle Mass Index and All-Cause Mortality Risk in Adults: A Systematic Review and Meta-Analysis of Prospective Cohort Studies," PLOS ONE 18, no. 6 (2023): e0286745, https://doi.org/10.1371/journal.pone.0286745.

147   Chun-Kit Law et al., "Physical Exercise Attenuates Cognitive Decline and Reduces Behavioural Problems in People with Mild Cognitive Impairment and Dementia: A Systematic Review," Journal of Physiotherapy 66, no. 1 (2020): 9-18, https://doi.org/10.1016/j.jphys.2019.11.014.

148   Matthew Thorpe, "How to Manage and Treat Muscle Loss from Sarcopenia Due to Aging," Healthline, published May 25, 2017, last modified April 14, 2025, https://www.healthline.com/nutrition/sarcopenia.

149   Barbara Strasser and Martin Burtscher, "Survival of the Fittest: VO2max, a Key Predictor of Longevity?," Frontiers in Bioscience (Landmark Edition) 23, no. 8 (2018): 1505-16, https://doi.org/10.2741/4657.

150   Prathiyankara Shailendra et al., "Weight Training and Risk of All-Cause, Cardiovascular Disease and Cancer Mortality among Older Adults," International Journal of Epidemiology 53, no. 3 (2024): dyae074, https://doi.org/10.1093/ije/dyae074.

151   Uwe Proske and Simon C. Gandevia, "The Proprioceptive Senses: Their Roles in Signaling Body Shape, Body Position and Movement, and Muscle Force," Physiological Reviews 92, no. 4 (2012): 1651-1697, https://doi.org/10.1152/physrev.00048.2011.

152   Kyle Mandsager et al., "Association of Cardiorespiratory Fitness With Long-term Mortality Among Adults Undergoing Exercise Treadmill Testing," JAMA Network Open 1, no. 6 (2018): e183605, https://doi.org/10.1001/jamanetworkopen.2018.3605.

153   Garmin Ltd., "VO2 Max. Standard Ratings," fēnix 7 Standard/Solar/Pro Series Owner's Manual, August 2025, https://www8.garmin.com/manuals/webhelp/GUID-C001C335-A8EC-4A41-AB0E-BAC434259F92/EN-US/GUID-1FBCCD9E-19E1-4E4C-BD60-1793B5B97EB3.html.

154   Eric V. Neufeld et al., "Heart Rate Acquisition and Threshold-Based Training Increases Oxygen Uptake at Metabolic Threshold in Triathletes: A Pilot Study," International Journal of Exercise Science 12, no. 2 (2019): 144-154, https://doi.org/10.70252/HNHZ4958.

155   Andrew P. Bacon et. al, "VO2max Trainability and High Intensity Interval Training in Humans: A Meta-Analysis," PLOS ONE 8, no. 9 (2013): e73182, https://doi.org/10.1371/journal.pone.0073182.

156   Lars Larsson et al., "Sarcopenia: Aging-Related Loss of Muscle Mass and Function," Physiological Reviews 99, no. 1 (2019): 427-511, https://doi.org/10.1152/physrev.00061.2017.

157   Richard W. Bohannon, "Grip Strength: An Indispensable Biomarker for Older Adults," Clinical Interventions in Aging 14 (2019): 1681-1691, https://doi.org/10.2147/CIA.S194543.

158   Joseph Bernstein et al., "Estimating Median Survival Following Hip Fracture Among Geriatric Females: (100 − Patient Age) ÷ 4," Cureus 14, no. 6 (2022): e26299, https://doi.org/10.7759/cureus.26299.

159   Ahmet Aslan, Tolga Atay, and Nevres Hürriyet Aydoğan, "Risk Factors for Mortality and Survival Rates in Elderly Patients Undergoing Hemiarthroplasty for Hip Fracture," Acta Orthopaedica et Traumatologica Turcica 54, no. 2 (2020): 138-143, https://doi.org/10.5152/j.aott.2020.02.298.

160   Lawrence Hayes, "What the Strength of Your Grip Can Tell You about Your Overall Health," The Conversation, May 19, 2025, https://theconversation.com/what-the-strength-of-your-grip-can-tell-you-about-your-overall-health-256271.

161   The McFarlands (@the.mcfarlands), "Aging in Perspective," TikTok video, March 15, 2024, https://www.tiktok.com/t/ZTrQSr7mF/.

162   Marian L. Tupy and Ronald Bailey, "Life Expectancy is Rising," Human Progress, March 1, 2023, https://humanprogress.org/trends/life-expectancy-is-rising/.

163   Amanda Ruggeri, "Do We Really Live Longer Than Our Ancestors?," BBC Future, October 2, 2018, https://www.bbc.com/future/article/20181002-how-long-did-ancient-people-live-life-span-versus-longevity.

164   Matthew Pearce et al., "Association Between Physical Activity and Risk of Depression: A Systematic Review and Meta-analysis," JAMA Psychiatry 79, no. 6 (2022): 550, https://doi.org/10.1001/jamapsychiatry.2022.0609.

165   Pearce et al., "Association Between Physical Activity," 550.

166   Tracy Burrows et al., "Effectiveness of Dietary Interventions in Mental Health Treatment: A Rapid Review of Reviews," Nutrition & Dietetics 79, no. 3 (2022): 279-290, https://doi.org/10.1111/1747-0080.12754.

167   Michael Noetel et al., "Effect of Exercise for Depression: Systematic Review and Network Meta-Analysis of Randomised Controlled Trials," BMJ 384 (2024): e075847, https://doi.org/10.1136/bmj-2023-075847.

168   University of South Australia. "Exercise More Effective Than Medicines to Manage Mental Health." February 24, 2023. https://www.unisa.edu.au/media-centre/Releases/2023/exercise-more-effective-than-medicines-to-manage-mental-health/.

169   Matthew Pearce et al., "Association Between Physical Activity and Risk of Depression: A Systematic Review and Meta-analysis," JAMA Psychiatry 79, no. 6 (2022): 550-59, https://doi.org/10.1001/jamapsychiatry.2022.0609.

170   Tracy Burrows et al., "Effectiveness of Dietary Interventions in Mental Health Treatment: A Rapid Review of Reviews," Nutrition & Dietetics 79, no. 3 (2022): 279-290, https://doi.org/10.1111/1747-0080.12754.

171   Noetel et al., "Effect of Exercise for Depression,"
        e075847.

172   Joshua E. Curtiss et al., "Cognitive-Behavioral Treat-
        ments for Anxiety and Stress-Related Disorders," Focus
        (American Psychiatric Publishing) 19, no. 2 (2021): 184-
        89, https://doi.org/10.1176/appi.focus.20200045.

173   Mutsuhiro Nakao et al., "Cognitive-Behavioral Therapy
        for Management of Mental Health and Stress-Related
        Disorders: Recent Advances in Techniques and Technol-
        ogies," BioPsychoSocial Medicine 15, no. 1 (2021): 16,
        https://doi.org/10.1186/s13030-021-00219-w.

174   Suma P. Chand, Daniel P. Kuckel, and Martin R. Hueck-
        er, "Cognitive Behavior Therapy," in StatPearls (Treasure
        Island, FL: StatPearls Publishing, 2025), last modified
        May 23, 2023, https://www.ncbi.nlm.nih.gov/books/
        NBK470241/.

175   Jenny Rosendahl, Cameron T. Alldredge, and Antonia
        Haddenhorst, "Meta-analytic Evidence on the Efficacy
        of Hypnosis for Mental and Somatic Health Issues: A
        20-Year Perspective," Frontiers in Psychology 14 (2024),
        https://doi.org/10.3389/fpsyg.2023.1330238.

176   Keara E. Valentine et al., "The Efficacy of Hypnosis as a
        Treatment for Anxiety: A Meta-Analysis," International
        Journal of Clinical and Experimental Hypnosis 67, no. 3
        (2019): 336-63, https://doi.org/10.1080/00207144.2019.1
        613863.

177   Donato Giuseppe Leo, Simon S. Keller, and Riccar-
        do Proietti, "'Close Your Eyes and Relax': The Role of
        Hypnosis in Reducing Anxiety, and Its Implications for
        the Prevention of Cardiovascular Diseases," Frontiers in
        Psychology 15 (2024): 1411835, https://doi.org/10.3389/
        fpsyg.2024.1411835.

178   Bessel A. van der Kolk et al., "A Randomized Con-
        trolled Study of Neurofeedback for Chronic PTSD,"
        PLOS ONE 11, no. 12 (2016): e0166752, https://doi.
        org/10.1371/journal.pone.0166752.

179   Martijn Arns et al., "Efficacy of Neurofeedback Treat-
        ment in ADHD: The Effects on Inattention, Impulsivity
        and Hyperactivity: A Meta-Analysis," Clinical EEG and
        Neuroscience 40, no. 3 (2009): 180-189, https://doi.
        org/10.1177/155005940904000311.

180   Zheng Xia et al., "Uncovering the Power of Neurofeed-
        back: A Meta-analysis of Its Effectiveness in Treating
        Major Depressive Disorders," Cerebral Cortex 34, no.
        6 (2024): bhae252, https://doi.org/10.1093/cercor/
        bhae252.

181   Or Dezachyo et al., "Intrinsic Functional Connectivity
        of the Anterior Cingulate Cortex Is Associated with
        Tolerance to Distress," eNeuro 8, no. 5 (2021): ENEU-
        RO.0277-21.2021, https://doi.org/10.1523/ENEU-
        RO.0277-21.2021.

182   Benny Voncken, "What Is Askesis? Understanding the
        Stoic Meaning and Practice," Via Stoica, accessed De-
        cember 23, 2025, https://viastoica.com/what-is-askesis/.

183   Benny Voncken, "How to Practice Stoic Voluntary
        Discomfort," Via Stoica, accessed December 23, 2025,
        https://viastoica.com/how-to-practice-stoic-volun-
        tary-discomfort/.

184   Emily C. Willroth et al., "Well-Being and Cognitive
        Resilience to Dementia-Related Neuropathology," Psy-
        chological Science 34, no. 3 (2022): 283-97, https://doi.
        org/10.1177/09567976221119828.

185   Liz Mineo, "Good Genes Are Nice, but Joy Is Better,"
        Harvard Gazette, April 11, 2017, https://news.harvard.
        edu/gazette/story/2017/04/over-nearly-80-years-har-
        vard-study-has-been-showing-how-to-live-a-healthy-
        and-happy-life/.

186   Robert J. Waldinger and Marc S. Schulz, "What's Love
        Got to Do with It? Social Functioning, Perceived Health,
        and Daily Happiness in Married Octogenarians," Psy-
        chology and Aging 25, no. 2 (2010): 422-431, https://
        doi.org/10.1037/a0019087.

187   Fishers Health Department, "Loneliness Is More
        Dangerous Than Smoking 15 Cigarettes A Day," April
        9, 2024, https://health.fishersin.gov/loneliness-is-more-
        dangerous-than-smoking-15-cigarettes-a-day/.

188   Nicholas Pimlott, "The Ministry of Loneliness," Canadi-
        an Family Physician 64, no. 3 (2018): 166, https://pmc.
        ncbi.nlm.nih.gov/articles/PMC5851382/.

189   Jeffrey A. Hall and Andy J. Merolla, "Connecting Every-
        day Talk and Time Alone to Global Well-Being," Human
        Communication Research 46, no. 1 (2020): 86-111,
        https://doi.org/10.1093/hcr/hqz014.

190   Christopher Bergland, "Social Nourishment + Re-
        storative Solitude = Human Thriving," The Athlete's
        Way (blog), Psychology Today, December 25, 2019,
        https://www.psychologytoday.com/au/blog/the-ath-
        letes-way/201912/social-nourishment-restorative-soli-
        tude-human-thriving.

191   Minakshi Biswas, Shu Chang, and Edward A. Gill,
        "Coronary Artery Calcium Scoring: A Brief Update
        and Look to the Future," LipidSpin, National Lipid
        Association, 2018, https://www.lipid.org/lipid-spin/pot-
        pourri-2018/coronary-artery-calcium-scoring-brief-up-
        date-and-look-future.

192   Biswas, Chang, and Gill, "Coronary Artery Calcium
        Scoring."

193   Jeffrey Xia, Kinan Bachour, Abdul-Rahman M. Sulei-
        man, Jacob S. Roberts, Sammy Sayed, and Geoffrey W.
        Cho, "Enhancing Coronary Artery Plaque Analysis via
        Artificial Intelligence-Driven Cardiovascular Computed
        Tomography," Therapeutic Advances in Cardiovascular
        Disease 18 (2024): 17539447241303399, https://doi.
        org/10.1177/17539447241303399.

194   CardioSmart News, "Half of Patients with Ideal Cho-
        lesterol Have Underlying Heart Risks," CardioSmart,
        American College of Cardiology, December 14, 2017,
        https://www.cardiosmart.org/news/2017/12/half-of-
        patients-with-ideal-cholesterol-have-underlying-heart-
        risks.

195   Leticia Fernández-Friera et al., "Normal LDL-Choles-
       terol Levels Are Associated with Subclinical Athero-
       sclerosis in the Absence of Risk Factors," Journal of the
       American College of Cardiology 70, no. 24 (2017): 2979,
       https://doi.org/10.1016/j.jacc.2017.10.024.

196   Erin Bryant, "Study Reveals How APOE4 Gene May In-
       crease Risk for Dementia," National Institute on Aging,
       March 16, 2021, https://www.nia.nih.gov/news/study-
       reveals-how-apoe4-gene-may-increase-risk-dementia.

197   Amanda M. Di Battista, Nicolette M. Heinsinger, and
       G. William Rebeck, "Alzheimer's Disease Genetic Risk
       Factor APOE-ε4 Also Affects Normal Brain Function,"
       Current Alzheimer Research 13, no. 11 (2016): 1200-
       1207, https://doi.org/10.2174/1567205013666160401115
       127.

198   "Genetics of Dementia," Practical Neurology, June 17,
       2021, https://practicalneurology.com/diseases-diagno-
       ses/alzheimer-disease-dementias/genetics-of-demen-
       tia/31803/.

199   Grzegorz Sienski et al., "APOE4 Disrupts Intracellu-
       lar Lipid Homeostasis in Human iPSC-Derived Glia,"
       Science Translational Medicine 13, no. 583 (2021):
       eaaz4564, https://doi.org/10.1126/scitranslmed.aaz4564.

200   Sienski et al., "APOE4 Disrupts Intracellular Lipid Ho-
       meostasis," eaaz4564.

201   David Brent, Nadine Melhem, and Gustavo Turecki,
       "Pharmacogenomics of Suicidal Events," Pharma-
       cogenomics 11, no. 6 (2010): 793-807, https://doi.
       org/10.2217/pgs.10.64.

202   Melissa D. Klein et al., "Clinical Utility of CYP2C19
       Genotyping to Guide Antiplatelet Therapy in Patients
       With an Acute Coronary Syndrome or Undergoing
       Percutaneous Coronary Intervention," Arteriosclerosis,
       Thrombosis, and Vascular Biology 39, no. 4 (2019): 647-
       52, https://doi.org/10.1161/ATVBAHA.118.311963.

203   "The Cost of Sequencing a Human Genome," National Human Genome Research Institute, last modified November 1, 2021, https://www.genome.gov/about-genomics/fact-sheets/Sequencing-Human-Genome-cost.

204   Talon Abernathy, "Costs of Common Prenatal Tests," ValuePenguin, August 29, 2025, https://www.valuepenguin.com/costs-common-prenatal-tests.

205   Canadian Agency for Drugs and Technologies in Health, Non-invasive Prenatal Testing: A Review of the Cost Effectiveness and Guidelines (Ottawa, ON: Canadian Agency for Drugs and Technologies in Health, 2014), https://www.ncbi.nlm.nih.gov/books/NBK274056/.

206   Rose McDermott et al., "Monoamine Oxidase A Gene (MAOA) Predicts Behavioral Aggression Following Provocation," Proceedings of the National Academy of Sciences 106, no. 7 (2009): 2118, https://doi.org/10.1073/pnas.0808376106.

207   Judit Diószegi, Erand Llanaj, and Róza Ádány, "Genetic Background of Taste Perception, Taste Preferences, and Its Nutritional Implications: A Systematic Review," Frontiers in Genetics 10 (2019): 1272, https://doi.org/10.3389/fgene.2019.01272.

208   S. Sanchez-Roige, J. C. Gray, J. MacKillop, C.-H. Chen, and A. A. Palmer, "The Genetics of Human Personality," Genes, Brain and Behavior 17, no. 3 (2018): e12439, https://doi.org/10.1111/gbb.12439.

209   Howard J. Edenberg and Tatiana Foroud, "Genetics and Alcoholism," Nature Reviews Gastroenterology & Hepatology 10, no. 8 (2013): 487-94, https://doi.org/10.1038/nrgastro.2013.86.

210   David A. Kalmbach et al., "Genetic Basis of Chronotype in Humans: Insights From Three Landmark GWAS," Sleep 40, no. 2 (2017): zsw048, https://doi.org/10.1093/sleep/zsw048.

211   Iman Kassam, "CYP1A2: It's Not Just the 'Caffeine
       Gene,'" DNALabs, accessed December 24, 2025, https://
       dnalabs.ca/cyp1a2-its-not-just-the-caffeine-gene/.

212   Mitzi M. Gonzales et al., "Senolytic Therapy to Mod-
       ulate the Progression of Alzheimer's Disease (SToMP-
       AD): A Pilot Clinical Trial," The Journal of Prevention
       of Alzheimer's Disease 9, no. 1 (2022): 22-29, https://
       doi.org/10.14283/jpad.2021.62.

213   Kenneth Lou, "The 11 Biomarkers Bryan Johnson
       Tracks to Live Longer (and Why You Should Too)," Mito
       Health (blog), accessed December 24, 2025, https://mi-
       tohealth.com/blog/the-11-biomarkers-bryan-johnson-
       tracks-to-live-longer.

214   Charlotte Alter, "Bryan Johnson's Quest for Im-
       mortality," Time, September 20, 2023, https://time.
       com/6315607/bryan-johnsons-quest-for-immortality/.

215   Sandeep Palakodeti, MD MPH (@DrDeepMD),
       "Was just on a great small group discussion with
       @bryan_johnson," X (formerly Twitter), Janu-
       ary 10, 2025, 5:02 p.m., https://x.com/drdeepmd/
       status/1877838445181362386?s=46&t=HB-
       cZyR9QBlAMGHXaO54_Iw

216   Shameek Rakshit et al., "The Burden of Medical Debt in
       the United States," Peterson-KFF Health System Tracker,
       February 12, 2024, https://www.healthsystemtracker.
       org/brief/the-burden-of-medical-debt-in-the-united-
       states/.

217   Lunna Lopes et al., "Health Care Debt In The U.S.: The
       Broad Consequences Of Medical And Dental Bills,"
       KFF, June 16, 2022, https://www.kff.org/health-costs/
       kff-health-care-debt-survey/.

218   U.S. Bureau of Labor Statistics. "Medical Care Premiums
       in the United States, March 2023." Last modified April
       11, 2024. https://www.bls.gov/ebs/factsheets/medical-
       care-premiums-in-the-united-states.htm.

219   U.S. Bureau of Labor Statistics, "Medical Care Premiums."

220   Helen Santoro, "Health Insurers' $371 Billion Windfall," The Lever, December 11, 2024, https://www.levernews. com/health-insurers-371-billion-windfall.

221   Fred Pennic, "Almost 4 in 5 Physicians Employed By Hospitals, Health Systems, Corporate Entities," HIT Consultant, April 12, 2024, https://hitconsultant.net/2024/04/12/almost-4-in-5-physicians-employed-by-hospitals-health-systems-corporate-entities/.

222   Aaron Young et al., "FSMB Census of Licensed Physicians in the United States, 2024," Journal of Medical Regulation 111, no. 2 (2025): 7-17, https://doi.org/10.30770/2572-1852-111.2.7.

223   Rob Lott, "Does UnitedHealthcare Pay Optum Providers Differently? w/ Dan Arnold," November 18, 2025, in Health Affairs Podcast, podcast, 25:00, https://doi.org/10.1377/hp20251113.858460.

224   American Medical Association, "RVS Update Committee (RUC)," last modified November 17, 2025, https://www.ama-assn.org/about/rvs-update-committee-ruc/rvs-update-committee-ruc.

225   Phillip L. Swagel, The Prices That Commercial Health Insurers and Medicare Pay for Hospitals' and Physicians' Services (Washington, DC: Congressional Budget Office, January 2022), https://www.cbo.gov/publication/57778.

226   Office of Disease Prevention and Health Promotion, "Healthy People 2030," U.S. Department of Health and Human Services, accessed December 25, 2025, https://odphp.health.gov/healthypeople.

227   Robert Lufkin, Lies I Taught in Medical School: How Conventional Medicine Is Making You Sicker and What You Can Do to Save Your Own Life (BenBella Books, 2024), p. 81.

228   Lufkin, Lies I Taught in Medical School, p. 157.

229   Lufkin, Lies I Taught in Medical School, p. 189.

230   Lufkin, Lies I Taught in Medical School, pp. 5-7.

231   Atul Bali and Roopa Naik, "The Impact of a Vegan Diet
           on Many Aspects of Health: The Overlooked Side of
           Veganism," Cureus 15, no. 2 (2023): e35148, https://doi.
           org/10.7759/cureus.35148.

232   Edyta Łuszczki et al., "Vegan Diet: Nutritional Compo-
           nents, Implementation, and Effects on Adults' Health,"
           Frontiers in Nutrition 10 (2023): 1294497, https://doi.
           org/10.3389/fnut.2023.1294497.

233   Łuszczki et al., "Vegan Diet."

234   Dimitra Rafailia Bakaloudi et al., "Intake and Adequacy
           of the Vegan Diet: A Systematic Review of the Evi-
           dence," Clinical Nutrition 40, no. 5 (2021): 3503, https://
           doi.org/10.1016/j.clnu.2020.11.035.

235   Anshika Malhotra and Ankita Lakade, "Analytical Re-
           view on Nutritional Deficiencies in Vegan Diets: Risks,
           Prevention, and Optimal Strategies," Journal of the
           American Nutrition Association 44, no. 6 (2025): 545-
           555, https://doi.org/10.1080/27697061.2025.2461218.

236   Eliška Selinger et al., "Evidence of a Vegan Diet for
           Health Benefits and Risks – an Umbrella Review of
           Meta-Analyses of Observational and Clinical Studies,"
           Critical Reviews in Food Science and Nutrition 63, no.
           29 (2023): 9926-36, https://doi.org/10.1080/10408398.20
           22.2075311.

237   Cleveland Clinic, "Zinc Deficiency," Cleveland Clinic,
           last reviewed February 11, 2025, https://my.cleveland-
           clinic.org/health/diseases/zinc-deficiency.

238   Isabel Iguacel et al., "Veganism, Vegetarianism, Bone
           Mineral Density, and Fracture Risk: A Systematic
           Review and Meta-Analysis," Nutrition Reviews 77, no.
           1 (January 2019): 1-18, https://doi.org/10.1093/nutrit/
           nuy045.

239   Isabel Iguacel, Inge Huybrechts, Luis A. Moreno, and Nathalie Michels, "Vegetarianism and Veganism Compared with Mental Health and Cognitive Outcomes: A Systematic Review and Meta-Analysis," Nutrition Reviews 79, no. 4 (2021): 361-81, https://doi.org/10.1093/nutrit/nuaa030.

240   Bakaloudi et al., "Intake and Adequacy of the Vegan Diet," 3510.

241   Christine Richmond, "Signs You're Not Getting Enough Protein," WebMD, August 30, 2024, https://www.webmd.com/diet/ss/slideshow-not-enough-protein-signs.

242   Bakaloudi et al., "Intake and Adequacy of the Vegan Diet," 3510.

243   Cleveland Clinic, "Iodine Deficiency: Symptoms, Causes, Treatment & Prevention," Cleveland Clinic, last modified July 7, 2022, https://my.clevelandclinic.org/health/diseases/23417-iodine-deficiency.

244   Malgorzata A. Desmond, Mary S. Fewtrell, and Jonathan C. K. Wells, "Plant-Based Diets in Children: Secular Trends, Health Outcomes, and a Roadmap for Urgent Practice Recommendations and Research—A Systematic Review," Nutrients 16, no. 5 (2024): 723, https://doi.org/10.3390/nu16050723.